Handbuch der Urologie
Encyclopedia of Urology

V/1

Supplement

Editores

L. Andersson R. F. Gittes W. E. Goodwin
W. Lutzeyer E. Zingg

Diagnostic Radiology

Supplement

Radionuclides in Urology
Urological Ultrasonography
Percutaneous Puncture Nephrostomy

By

L. Andersson I. Fernström G.R. Leopold
J. U. Schlegel L. B. Talner

Edited by

L. Andersson

With 88 Figures

Springer-Verlag Berlin Heidelberg New York 1977

ISBN-13: 978-3-642-66466-3 e-ISBN-13: 978-3-642-66464-9
DOI:10.1007/978-3-642-66464-9

Library of Congress Cataloging in Publication Data: (Revised) Main entry under title: Handbuch der Urologie. Encyclopedia of urology. Vols. published after 1964 have imprint: Berlin, New York, Springer-Verlag. Includes bibliographies. Contents: 1. Anatomie und Embryologie, von K. Conrad et al. 1969. – 2. Physiologie und pathologische Physiologie, von B. Fey et al. 1965. – 3. Symptomatologie und Untersuchung von Blut, Harn und Genitalsekreten, von K. Hinsberg et al. 1960. [etc.]
1. Urology – Collected works. I. Alken, Carl Erich, 1912– ed. II. Title: Encyclopedia of urology. [DNLM: 1. Urologic diseases – Diagnosis. 2. Radioisotopes – Diagnostic use. 3. Ultrasonics – Diagnostic use. 4. Punctures. 5. Kidney pelvis – Surgery. WJ100 H237 Bd. 5 T. 1 Suppl.]
RC871.H28 616.6 58-4788

Preface

This book is a supplement to Volume V/1 in the present series, Diagnostic Radiology, published in 1962. Despite the relatively long period of time which has elapsed since its publication, that comprehensive volume is still essentially valid, even though further developments have of course occurred in certain fields.

In recent years the developments in nuclear medicine and ultrasonic techniques have led to a number of new methods of medical investigation, which, in different ways, complement diagnostic radiology. Functional disorders of the urinary tract can often be detected by means of radioisotopes. Since morphologic changes are almost always preceeded by functional disturbances, radionuclide techniques in many instances produce an earlier diagnosis than radiography. Disturbances of renal blood flow, slight ureteric obstruction, and ureteric reflux are examples of pathologic states which can be detected early by the γ scintillation camera.

Bone scans, i.e., imaging of the skeletal system using a radionuclide, are used extensively to diagnose bone metastases now that it has been demonstrated that such metastatic growths are identified both earlier and with greater accuracy by scintigraphy than by radiographic techniques.

Even though studies with the γ camera not only give a good idea of the renal blood flow and function but also visualize a renal mass, they are inferior to radiologic techniques and ultrasonography for the evaluation of the nature of the mass. Ultrasonography is a reliable method for the visualization of calculi in the urinary tract and for differentiating between a solid and a cystic renal mass; moreover, it is noninvasive. In the differential diagnosis of solid, space-occupying lesions of the kidney, nephroangiography is, however, the preferred technique.

Radionuclide studies and ultrasonography are by no means substitutes for radiographic techniques but rather, in certain situations, are complementary methods which yield equivalent or superior information, at the same time putting less strain on the patient, and are less expensive, once the equipment has been acquired. Radionuclide studies and ultrasonography both undoubtedly merit wider use in urologic diagnostics than they are given today. An outline of these methods and their application in the field of urology is given in this book.

Advances in modern radiographic television techniques have made it possible to perform not only angiographic examinations via percutaneous punctures but also certain operative procedures on deep tissues. Examples of this are the plugging of an aneurysm, or of arteries to an inoperable tumor, the extraction of calculi in the biliary or urinary tract, and the drainage of urine. This new operative principle involves considerably less strain on the patient than open surgery and therefore deserves wider use, although it requires special training of the operator. We consider the development of percutaneous puncture nephrostomy to be an advance of such significance as to justify a presentation of the method in this volume.

Stockholm, July 1977 L. Andersson

Contents

Radionuclides in Urology

J.U. SCHLEGEL

With 36 Figures

Urological Ultrasonography

G.R. LEOPOLD and L.B. TALNER

With 22 Figures

Percutaneous Puncture Nephrostomy

I. Fernström and L. Andersson

With 30 Figures

List of Contributors

Professor Dr. L. Andersson, Department of Urology, Karolinska sjukhuset, Stockholm, Sweden

Dr. I. Fernström, Department of Urology, Karolinska sjukhuset, Stockholm, Sweden

Professor Dr. G.R. Leopold, Section of Uroradiology, University of California, University Hospital, 225 West Dickinson Street, San Diego CA 92103/USA

Professor Dr. J.U. Schlegel, Chairman, Department of Urology, Tulane University School of Medicine, 1430 Tulane Avenue, New Orleans LA 70112/USA

Professor Dr. L.B. Talner, Head, Section of Uroradiology, University of California, University Hospital, 225 West Dickinson Street, San Diego CA 92103/USA

Radionuclides in Urology

J.U. SCHLEGEL

With 36 Figures

A. Introduction

Almost every area in diagnostic urology has been influenced by the explosive development of nuclear medicine. The list is long and impressive, and touches nearly every organ, not the least of which is the kidney. The urologist, however, cannot ignore the radionuclides as they can be applied to the diagnosis of lung metastasis, pulmonary infarcts, subphrenic abscess, liver metastasis, trauma, and a host of other pathologic conditions originating from, or having a bearing on, diseases of the genitourinary system. As BLAUFOX (1972) stated:

> It is unfortunate that many clinicians, who consider the use of radionuclides in nephrology, think only of the radiorenogram. The renogram, which achieved its greatest clinical acceptance shortly after its inception in 1955, has been greatly overemphasized in nuclear medicine. The procedure surely is useful clinically, but its greatest shortcoming has been the overenthusiastic application of renography by individuals attempting to achieve far-reaching diagnoses beyond the capability of a screening procedure. The continuing introduction of new methods of analysis and of controversy about the renogram have severely limited its credibility.

The evolution of the gamma scintillation camera has, however, changed all of this, and the application of this modality with available techniques for quantitation amounts to the clinical application of modern renal physiology. The noninvasiveness and lack of morbidity makes it a *sine qua non* in diagnostic urology, and its widespread use is likely just a matter of time.

Radiology as we know it today did not just happen. It is at this writing 80 years ago that roentgen rays were discovered, and the first attempt to perform intravenous pyelography dates back to 1923. The first shipment of radioisotopes for use in medicine was made on August 2, 1946, from Oak Ridge, a fallout of the wartime Manhattan Project. In 1952, diagnosis of renal disease was first attempted by OESER and BILLION, who measured excretion of ^{131}I-labeled sodium methramate from each kidney, and TAPLIN (1972) and coworkers first designed the radioisotope renogram in 1956. The present-day gamma scintillation camera has, however, only been available to the medical profession for less than 10 years, and the hardware and software which can be purchased today is of even more recent vintage.

The tremendous explosion in diagnostic nuclear medicine following World War II involving radiopharmaceuticals and instrumentation of a highly sophisticated nature has led to a knowledge gap which must be bridged if the urological patient is to benefit from this progress in modern medical technology. The average physician and specialist today has had very little exposure to and training in nuclear medicine, and it is imperative that this be corrected. The urologist to whom this text is primarily addressed should learn to be as conversant with nuclear medicine in urological diagnosis as he is with urological radiology. Only then can he appreciate what it can do for his patients. It is hoped that this text will help in this endeavor, but it should also be appreciated that urological nuclear medicine tomorrow may be a far cry from what it is today. However, only by knowing what it can do today can we help in shaping tomorrow.

In the following pages, we will try to describe the present state of the art as it involves various organs of interest to the urologist in clinical practice and in research. In our department we have used renal scintillation camera studies as a primary diagnostic tool in more than 20,000 patients, and find it indispensable in accuracy and dependability. Our experience in this area will be further detailed in a later section; here in the introductory remarks we want merely to emphasize that it is our firm conviction that the application of nuclear medicine to diagnostic urology is a boon to the patient and the urologist alike. It should further be added that the instrumentation, radiopharmaceuticals, and application are still in their infancy, and adulthood is going to be even more exciting. It is our feeling that if the urologist does not take advantage of this golden opportunity someone else will, and this may not serve the best interest of our patients or our profession.

B. Renal Clearances

Renal clearances have never gained wide acceptance in clinical medicine because of the difficulties entailed in serum and urine analysis and not the least because of the known problems inherent in accurate urine collections on a hospital ward. The emergence of radionuclides has, to some extent, minimized the analytical problems and in attempts to get away from the necessity of accurate urine collections, several other approaches to determination of renal function have come into at least limited use.

To use radionuclides for standard clearance methods, it is expected that such labeled compounds have identical, or at least similar, clearance to the standards used in the past for determination of glomerular filtration rates, i.e., inulin, and for effective renal plasma flow, i.e., paraminohippuric acid.

Table 1. Radionuclides used for ERPF and GFR measurements

Measurement	Isotope	Compound
ERPF	^{125}I, ^{131}I	Iodohippurate
ERPF	^{131}I	Iodopyracet
GFR	^{125}I, ^{131}I	Iothalamate
GFR	^{131}I	Diatrizoate
GFR	^{125}I, ^{51}Cr	Inulin
GFR	^{57}Co	Vitamin B_{12} (cyanocobalamin)
GFR	^{51}Cr	EDTA
GFR	^{99m}Tc, ^{169}Yb, ^{113m}In, ^{140}La	DTPA

Attempts to do away with intravenous infusion to maintain constant serum levels have been made with intradermal injection of a small volume of high specific activity for determination of GFR as well as ERPF, but the method never seemed to gain widespread acceptance (Koss et al., 1965; Wisenbaugh et al., 1965). Although as previously stated, classical clearance techniques are not very useful in the clinical setting, they are nevertheless still important since the handling of various compounds with various labels by the normal as well as the diseased kidney must be known before one attempts to interpret results that may be misleading. A number of review articles as well as numerous studies concerning the use of radionuclides for determination of renal clearances are available; however, it should be added that utilizing spectrophotometers, it is relatively simple to determine GFR and ERPF simultaneously, thus obtaining information about filtration fraction.

To overcome the problem of timed urine collections, several investigators have recommended, and made use of, single injection clearance, analyzing in various ways the plasma disappearance curve (Blaufox, 1972).

Apart from clearance technique and plasma disappearance rate, renal blood flow can be determined by catheterization of the renal artery and vein, utilizing either extraction ratio, indicator dilution, or inert gas wash-out. $I^{133}Xe$ or ^{85}Kr both have been used to provide data on intrarenal distribution of blood flow. For more information concerning these techniques, the reader is referred to review articles by GRUNFELD et al. (1974) and BLAUFOX (1972).

C. Renal Function Studies with External Scintillation Probe

The first externally performed radionuclide test of individual kidney function was done in January, 1955, resulting in the first clinical application shortly thereafter. As has previously been alluded to, this technique, which has formed the basis in principle for today's much more sophisticated external counting devices, is probably of little use as a general clinical tool except perhaps in very specific areas, such as renal transplantation. Although a great deal of work in regard to analysis of the renogram has been done, principally by BROWN and BRITTON (1972), as well as by others, it appears that the utilization of an external probe with a single photocell is not practical for the usual clinical application when scintillation cameras are available and can eliminate some of the inherent problems by direct visualization. The external scintillation probe, however, is still a useful tool for many special applications as well as various types of renal function studies. An excellent review of the compartment analysis of the renogram and kinetics of ^{131}I labeled Hippuran, as well as the description of the normal renogram was recently published (BLAUFOX, 1972; WEDEEN and BLAUFOX, 1972).

A method for determination of renal clearance utilizing an external monitoring of plasma concentration was developed in the dog, utilizing Radiohippuran. The method requires no urine collection and adjusts the rate of isotope infusion to maintain a constant emission rate equal to the concurrent rate of renal extraction (GAGNON et al., 1972; and WAGGENKNECHT et al., 1971). This method sounds very ingenious and apparently gives quite an accurate evaluation of the effective renal plasma flow, but has of yet not been subjected to any exhaustive use in patients.

Renal scintillation scanning is today almost completely replaced by renal sequential imaging, although in many instances clinicians consider the terms identical. The scintillation scan is obtained by the mechanical movement of a scintillation probe over the large or small area it is desired to record radioactivity from, and then at the same time, obtain a mapping of its spatial distribution. Whether the scintillation probe is a gamma camera mechanically moved over the entire body to obtain, for instance, a skeletal scan, or whether it is a small scintillation probe moving in a preset pattern over the brain or renal area, scanning and especially total body scanning is still a very useful procedure. However, renal scanning is practically nonexistent today and has been replaced by scintillation imaging using a camera.

D. Renal and Urinary Tract Function Utilizing a Gamma Scintillation Camera

A noninvasive, rapid way to assess individual as well as total kidney function would be a tremendously useful tool dealing with many types of disease processes and possibly even in the seemingly healthy individual. The value of being able to assess individual renal function is not only of importance in dealing with diseases within the genitourinary system, but also in dealing with diseases of other organs where complications secondary to unsuspected renal disease may be minimized if proper assessment can be made prior to therapy. This naturally is true for many types of surgical procedures where fluid and electrolyte handling should be based upon knowledge of renal function, and where administration of drugs should take into consideration their elimination by the kidneys. Detection of possible iatrogenic damage to the ureters, bladder, or even the kidneys can be dealt with more readily and easily if preoperative or pretrauma knowledge of the urinary tract is at hand.

The determination of serum creatinine as well as BUN is clinically often used to assess any gross deterioration in kidney function, but it is well realized that this is indeed a gross evaluation, inasmuch as kidney function may be half of normal without any abnormalities being apparent with these serum determinations. In addition, there is no guarantee that a given patient has two normal kidneys, and although intravenous urography will supply morphologic information, it is well known to be a poor test for evaluation of kidney function.

The gamma scintillation camera with proper attachments for the quantitation of electronically tagged areas of interest can indeed provide the answers to all of these things, even though it certainly must be emphasized that detailed morphology can in no way compete with a properly performed roentgenogram, whether it be intravenous urogram, angiogram, nephrotomogram, or retrograde pyelogram. It should, however, be emphasized that morphologic changes usually occur secondary to functional changes, and it is exceedingly rare to find a totally normal scintillation camera study in the face of significant pathology. It can certainly not be denied that a small hypernephroma or transitional cell tumor as well as a silent stone may exist in the face of a normal scintillation camera study, i.e., normal gross morphology and normal function; but then such pathology can easily be missed also on routine screening by intravenous urography, and if there is no hematuria, there is little chance that such a patient would be subjected to a more detailed evaluation. If hematuria is present, we do not propose that the scintillation camera be used exclusively to rule out the presence of pathology, because this is a clear-cut indication for detailed radiologic evaluation. Such is obviously also the case if the scintillation camera study is abnormal; however, it is our considered opinion at this point that it is possible, with proper and available equipment, to obtain detailed information about the absolute functional integrity of the individual kidney as well as gross morphology in a matter of approximately 3 min with the injection of ^{131}I labeled Hippuran, with a radiation dose that is insignificant in the average individual with normal kidney function. To decrease the possible uptake of radioactive iodine to the thyroid, especially in the small child, the routine use of Lugol's solution is suggested, thus even further minimizing any possible radiation risk. With the latest developments within this area, it should be possible at least in any hospitalized patient to obtain an accurate assessment of the individual renal function as well as gross morphology within a period of time that is insignificant (3 min) and certainly be able to obtain much more valuable information than is obtainable by the usual routine electrocardiogram. If this indeed, as we suspect, will become a standard, the cost factor also becomes insignificant, since it, to a great extent, will be reduced to the cost of the radioisotopes with but a small fraction necessary for capitalizing the basic equipment. It is thus our intention in this presentation to first describe our experience in the routine use of the gamma scintillation camera for screening procedures in any urological patient, and then to discuss the developments that have resulted, before then going on to specific applications of the gamma scintillation camera for specific diagnostic approaches and dealing with specific disease entities.

Screening for renal and urinary tract diseases utilizing a gamma scintillation camera and ^{131}I Hippuran has been used by this author since 1968 and essentially is unchanged as originally described. It is based upon several components, the first of which is the percentage distribution of renal Radiohippuran uptake in the period of 1–2 min following the injection. The reason that we have used the interval of 1–2 min is, first, because the early uptake sometimes reflects on the right side some hepatic uptake which ordinarily is very minimal after the first 60 s. The second factor is due to the rapid excretion of Radiohippuran, but in the average individual no radioactivity has appeared in the renal collecting system before 2 min following the injection. Apart from the relative distribution of Radiohippuran between the two kidneys, which is indicative of relative renal blood flow, total renal blood flow is determined by recovering all urine at 30 min after the injection and determining the percentage return of the injected amount. This relates directly to total renal blood flow. Finally, a 60-s count is made over the bladder before and after urination at approximately 30 min following the injection, which allows calculation of the exact amount of residual urine, if any is present. The minute to minute count rates can be presented as a renal histogram, giving a graphic presentation similar to the renogram curve. It should, however, be pointed out that all the counts over the kidneys are derived by either electronically tagging the kidneys or setting zones of interest, excluding most areas outside the kidney. We have recently started to use background subtraction. However, this is not necessary in the average case, especially if the kidney function is within normal limits, but is primarily of use for determination of absolute count rates as we will describe later.

The patient should be in a state of adequate hydration and is usually given several cups of water immediately prior to the procedure. The purpose of this is to insure a reasonably brisk flow of urine, whereby a normal individual usually will have only a little radioactivity left in the collecting system by 30 min. A scintiphoto obtained over the kidneys at this time will insure, in conjunction with bladder counts after urination, that the 30-min return is indeed a return with no excessive amount of radionuclide remaining over the renal or bladder area. The patient is placed in the supine position with the camera underneath, and only rarely will the experienced technician encounter a situation where both kidneys are not covered by the crystal. Occasionally we have used a transmission image using a ^{57}Co disk which is placed above the patient and which allows ready visualization of the diaphragm and thus easy placement of the patient. Many other ways of using an anatomical landmark, including the possibility of labeling the kidneys with ^{197}Hg labeled Neohydrin, have been proposed, but we rarely find the need for any of these procedures in the average individual. To insure reproducability in count rates, the counting is started using a foot switch which is activated immediately following the completion of 2.5 ml i.v. containing the proper dose of the ^{131}I labeled Hippuran. The dose schedule is as follows:

Age 0–6 months	= 50 μCi
Age 6–24 months	=100 μCi
Age 24 months to 12 years	=200 μCi
Age 12 years and older	=300 μCi

When the appropriate dose has been calculated, the exact activity to be administered is then measured in a dose calibrator. Following intravenous injection of the radiopharmaceutical, the syringe is placed again in the dose calibrator and the remaining radioactivity is then subtracted from the originally measured dose, giving the exact dose injected.

All the raw data obtained is recorded on videotape and a 0–3 min scintiphoto is obtained to allow visual inspection of possible morphologic abnormalities. The equipment necessary for electronic tagging and quantitation need not be present in the location where the scintillation camera study is done, and we have for years analyzed data obtained on videotape from clinical and hospital facilities that do not have the equipment allowing quantitation within areas of interest. Any abnormality, except perhaps for renal tumors less than 2.5–3 cm in diameter and not causing any obstruction or decrease in kidney function, is detectable by this technique, and if urinalysis is an integral portion of this screening procedure, it is doubtful that any abnormalities would be missed which would not be missed by anything but the most sophisticated radiologic procedure. Although this approach appears useful in the large number of patients, there are situations where it is not useful, such as in patients who cannot void upon command, which particularly would be true for children under 2 years of age, as well as in situations where obstructive uropathy prevents an adequate determination of return in 30 min. In such patients, the technique as described will not allow accurate determination of total kidney function, although the relative renal blood flow still would be valid. Minor discrepancies in emptying may sometimes be obscured by diuresis and under such circumstances, the camera study in a state of dehydration may be preferable. This may be true in children with reflux, in some patients with renovascular hypertension, as well as in patients with lesser degrees of obstructive uropathy secondary to ureteral or renal calculi, transitional cell tumors, or inflammatory processes. For this reason, we have for several years attempted to try to determine not only relative renal blood flow but also absolute individual renal blood flow without the necessity for collection of urine or blood sampling.

The renal uptake of Radiohippuran determined by actual counting over the renal areas with background subtraction is a function of renal blood flow. In comparing renal function from individual to individual or in the same individual from time to time, only two factors seem to enter into this relationship, the first being that of renal blood flow, and the second being that of the renal distance from the crystal. The latter can be readily calculated on the basis of height and weight, as has been suggested by TAUXE and HUNT (1966), as well as by NORMAN (1972) and TØNNESEN et al. (1974).

Norman's regression equation for the mean depth of the two kidneys (Y) is

$$Y = 13.7 \text{ times } X + 0.5,$$

(X) being the weight–height ratio.

This data was obtained on autopsy material by pushing a needle from the center of the kidney backwards vertically on the skin surface. The equation obtained by TØNNESEN et al. (1974), was quite similar, and was obtained by ultrasonic measurements of the distance from the skin to the center of the kidney. There, regression for the left side was

$$Y = 13.2 \text{ times } X + 0.7,$$

and for the right,

$$Y = 13.3 \text{ times } X + 0.7.$$

SKRIPKA and SCHLEGEL (1975) in our department found that in people with normal kidney function, the renal photon flux, i.e., counts per channel, with background subtraction, had a straight linear relationship with the body surface area (Fig. 1).

Taking this data into consideration, we thus determine absolute renal blood flow by placing the syringe containing the radionuclides to be injected at a fixed distance above the collimator (Fig. 2).

Counting is recorded for 60 s, and counting over the kidneys after background subtraction for 60 s, at the 1–2 min period following the injection of Radiohippuran. Renal uptake is then expressed, after correction for kidney distance (multiplication with the square of the distance using the equation to which we have previously referred). This corrected kidney count is then expressed in relation to the original count present in the syringe (Fig. 3).

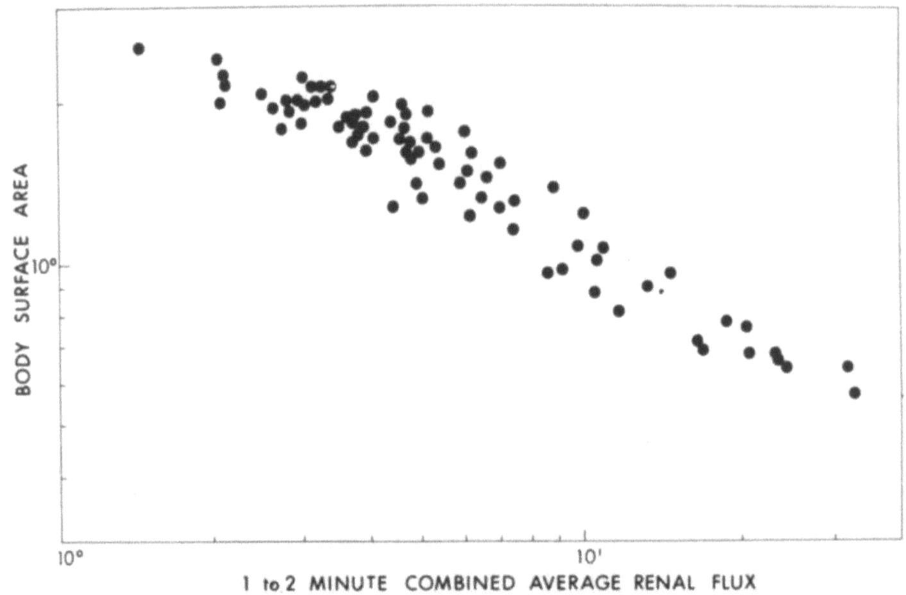

Fig. 1. Logarithmic presentation of counts per channel with background subtraction over renal area at 1–2 min after injection of ^{131}I labeled Hippuran versus log of body surface area. All individuals had normal renal function and it is seen that renal flux, i.e., counts per channel over kidney, is a function of the body surface area

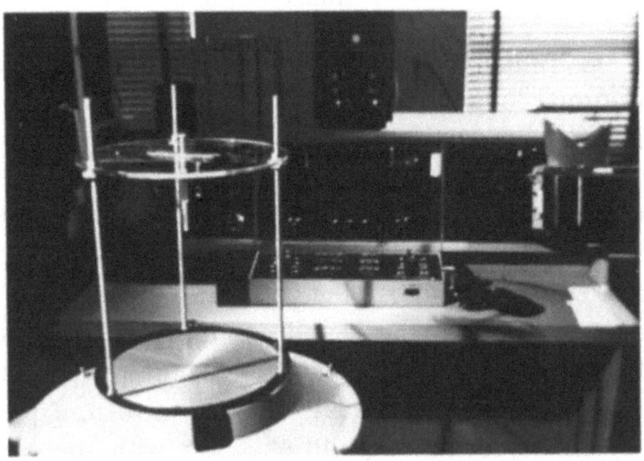

Fig. 2. Scaffold placed on face of gamma scintillation camera with syringe at fixed distance containing Radiohippuran to be injected intravenously. Controls for gamma camera with persistence scope and Polaroid camera are seen in background

$$\text{ERPF} = \frac{\text{1-2 MINUTE KIDNEY COUNT (LESS BACKGROUND)} \times Y^2}{\text{1 MINUTE COUNT OF RADIONUCLIDE INJECTED}} \times 100$$

$$x = \text{RATIO } \frac{\text{WEIGHT IN kg.}}{\text{HEIGHT IN cm.}}$$

$$Y = \text{KIDNEY DEPTH IN cm.} \qquad Y\ (\text{RIGHT}) = 13.3\,x + 0.7 \qquad Y\ (\text{LEFT}) = 13.2\,x + 0.7$$

Fig. 3. Effective renal plasma flow is calculated as 1–2 min kidney count with background subtraction multiplied with square of kidney depth times 100 and divided with 1 min count of radionuclide injected intravenously

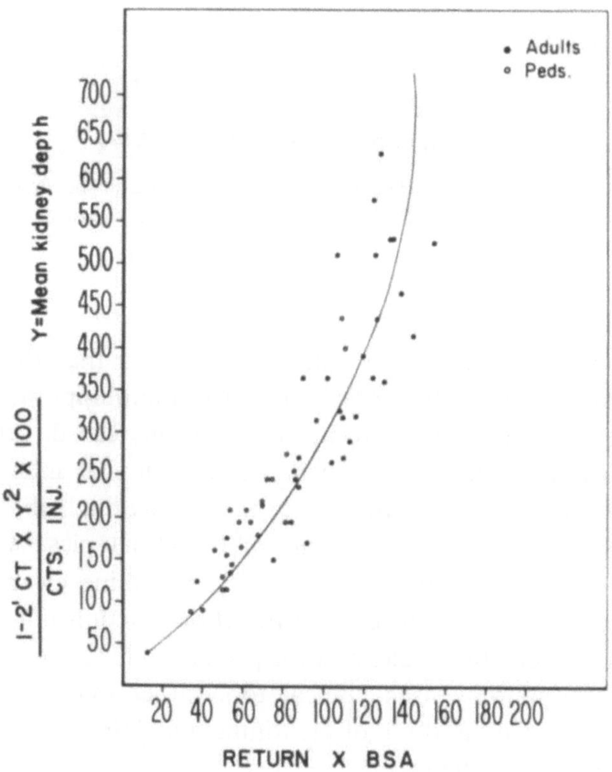

Fig. 4. Ratio of total renal counts multiplied with square of mean kidney depth and 100 divided with 1 min counts of radioactivity injected is plotted against 30 min return of Radiohippuran times body surface area

The combined or individual corrected renal count with background subtraction is then compared with kidney function as determined by return of the injected Radiohippuran, as illustrated in Figs. 4 and 5.

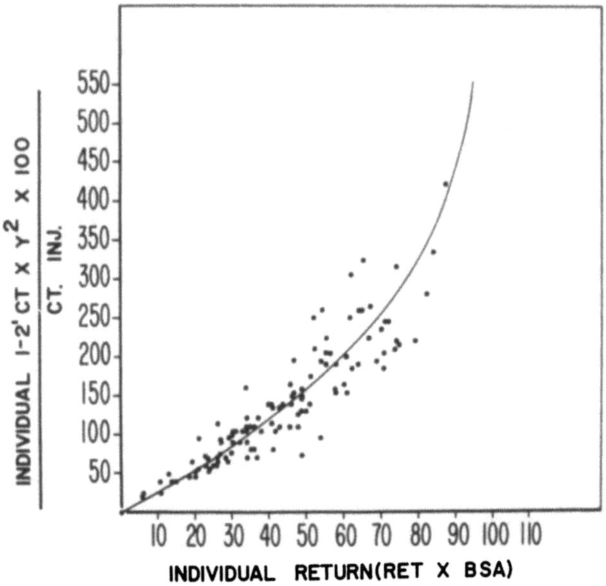

Fig. 5. Here individual renal counts are expressed as in Fig. 4, again showing good correlation with renal plasma flow as indicated by 30 min percentage return of Radiohippuran

As previously shown by the author and others that the return of Radiohippuran relates in a linear fashion to paraminohippurate clearance (Fig. 6) as well as creatinine clearance (Fig. 7), one can directly express the individual renal function as a clearance function, if such is desired, and thus a technique is available to express individual absolute renal blood flow without collection of urine or blood samples. Although in most instances this will correlate well with creatinine clearance, such will only hold true in cases where the filtration fraction is normal, and the comparison to creatinine clearance is primarily done for convenience, since this is a commonly used clinical tool rather than to attempt to indicate that the renal handling of creatinine and Hippuran is identical, which obviously is not the case.

The routine use of the gamma scintillation camera for determination of relative renal function has made use not only of ^{131}I-labeled Hippuran, but also several ^{99m}Tc compounds as well as ^{197}Hg-labeled Neohydrin. Various methods for determining the relative uptake by the two kidneys are used as far as instrumentation is concerned, from the split crystal to channel analyzers and table-top computers. It is, however, of considerable importance that accuracy is used for determination of individual

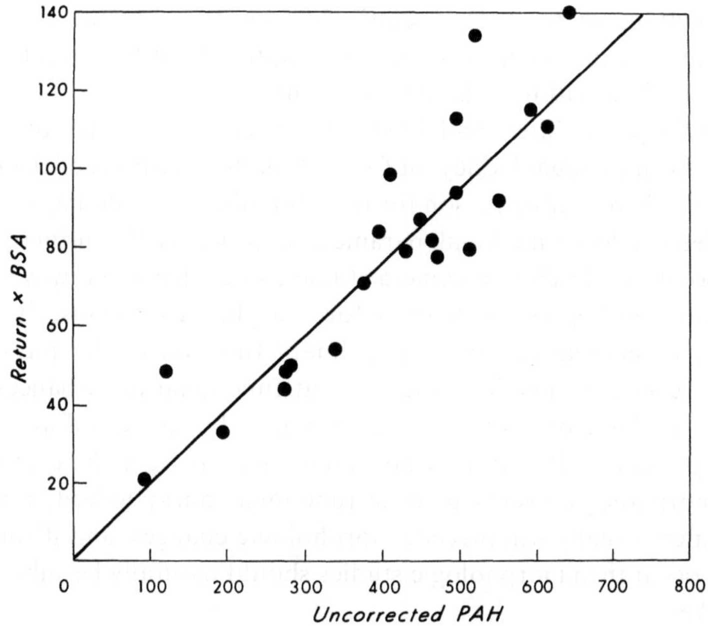

Fig. 6. The 30 min return of Radiohippuran times body surface area is here plotted against paraminohippurate clearance

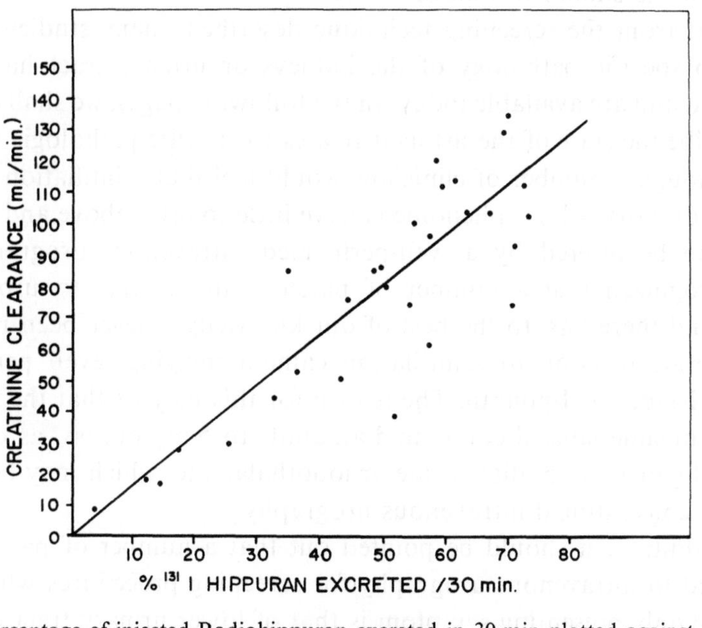

Fig. 7. Percentage of injected Radiohippuran excreted in 30 min plotted against creatinine clearance

renal function; to try to "eyeball" differences in uptake by the two kidneys may be just as misleading as attempting to utilize an intravenous urogram for evaluation of kidney function.

With the possibilities available for quantitation of uptake of radionuclides by the individual kidney, or for that matter, portions of the individual kidney, there is little reason for not obtaining accurate measurements that indeed reflect functional parameters, which is the primary virtue at this point of scintillation camera studies, since they in no way compete with proper radiologic evaluation for morphologic details. It should, however, be emphasized that the primary function of the physician is to preserve kidney function, and to treat functional disturbances rather than morphologic ones that occasionally may be congenital and of little or no significance. It is rare, if not impossible, to see a clinical situation where morphologic events precede functional ones; indeed, functional disturbances usually will precede morphologic changes, and if functional changes occur then morphologic studies should naturally be subsequently undertaken.

Although ^{131}I-labeled Hippuran is presently the most rapid and sensitive way of evaluating renal function, it must be admitted that ^{131}I is not the ideal radionuclide, but it is hoped that ^{123}I eventually will become available, providing the advantages of a pure gamma emitter with a short half-life similar to that of ^{99m}Tc.

Apart from the screening technique described, many studies as they relate to specific pathology of the kidneys or urinary tract have been described and are available today. In the following pages, we shall attempt to describe the state of the art as it relates to specific pathologic entities, and although a number of clinicians would feel that scintillation camera studies for morphologic phenomena have little to offer above and beyond what can be offered by a well-performed intravenous urogram, it is well recognized that a number of patients are allergic to urographic media and there has, to the best of our knowledge, never been reported any allergic reaction to scintillation camera imaging, even performed with ^{131}I-labeled Hippuran. The reason for this may be that the amount of radionuclide-labeled compound amounts to 5 mg or less, as opposed to 18–20 g or more of diatrizoate or iodothalamate, which may be necessary for conventional intravenous urography.

In addition, it should be pointed out that a number of patients are subjected to intravenous urography for screening procedures where perhaps the only presenting symptom is that of lower urinary tract obstruction. It is not an uncommon experience to see reports on, or to read, intravenous urograms where morphologic details leave a lot to be desired and where the interpretation often amounts to the description of various things that cannot be seen along with a conclusion like "probably normal," where a proper description should be that it is not diagnostic.

It is our experience that approximately 50% of routinely performed intravenous urograms for screening procedures are basically nondiagnostic and serve less of a useful purpose for evaluation of total and individual renal function than does a properly performed quantitative renal scintillation camera study. It is our considered opinion that intravenous urography is a superb technique for demonstrating, first and foremost, morphology of the collecting system, with a possible initial nephrogram to demonstrate the functioning renal mass, but it gives only a very gross and sometimes distorted evaluation of the kidney function, since most radiographic media are handled only by filtration. The gamma scintillation camera studies, especially utilizing Radiohippuran, give poor morphology but a superb evaluation of the individual renal blood flow if proper quantitation is utilized to obtain the maximum benefit which can be derived.

Finally, for renal mass evaluation, whether it is functioning or not, ultrasonography appears to be the tool of choice, and consequently one cannot look at one diagnostic tool as being superior to the other, but rather look at all diagnostic procedures for their proper roles and proper combination in making a diagnosis in a given situation. It should be further emphasized here that the least invasive techniques, such as the use of radionuclides or ultrasound, should preferably precede more invasive techniques, and in many instances may make the latter unnecessary. This would then reserve the more invasive techniques for precise evaluation of unexplained problems. The information obtained by the preliminary isotopic or sonographic studies may then be helpful in the broader understanding of the more invasive procedures. The collective use of the information thus obtained should lower the number of nondiagnostic procedures, partly because the work load may be more appropriately adjusted to individuals where it truly is indicated.

E. Renal Failure

The challenge to the clinician encountering a patient with azotemia or a urine volume which is below 500 ml in 24 h is an important one. Acute renal failure may be due to pathology that involved the blood supply to the kidney (considered prerenal) or it may be due to renal disease either from nephrotoxic agents or parenchymal disease, and last but not least, the cause may be postrenal, involving any obstructive uropathy stretching from the renal pelvis to the urethral meatus.

Chronic renal failure may entail the same pathologic entities and depending upon the degree of chronicity, it may be correctable, or it may have reached a point beyond repair. Since some of the problems entailed may be correctable, it obviously is of tremendous importance to make as early a diagnosis as possible, and it may be equally important to prognosticate so that proper consideration can be given, taking into account the individual patient as well as the underlying disease. Although it is obvious that many procedures can be valuable in ascertaining the proper information in such patients, including various radiologic examinations, it is equally well appreciated that intravenous urography in an azotemic patient is often, except in acute obstruction, of little or no help, and retrograde pyelography carries, especially in such patients, an increased morbidity which, in situations of nonobstructive uropathy, may be highly undesirable.

The use of radionuclides can be very helpful as an initial procedure since it is noninvasive, non-toxic, rapid, and quite simple. In a majority of cases, morphologic as well as functional information can be obtained. REBA et al. (1974), state that one of the main uses of nuclear medicine procedures in patients with renal failure is the determination of kidney size. They further state that mercury scanning frequently is successful, even if the BUN is in the range of 40–100 mg-%, but it is rarely successful if these levels exceed 100 mg-%. These authors recommend the use of radiolabeled chelates which are true glomerular substances and therefore not metabolized, sequestered, or excreted except by the kidneys. These substances will be distributed only within the extracellular space and after filtration within the kidney tubules. The visualization of the kidneys would be secondary to any water reabsorption of the filtered material so that the high photon emitting radionuclides will achieve renal visualization. The authors feel that these substances will make it possible to more readily identify renal structure in instances of renal insufficiency, particularly helpful in situations when the excretory urogram fails to visualize or is poorly visualized. If the renal function, according to these authors, is impaired, and prompt excretion and localization of the radionuclide is delayed, the mercury becomes bound to secondary sites of sulfhydryl binding such as the liver, so that in uremia, there seems to be a marked increase in hepatic localization, with excretion subsequently into the gastrointestinal tract, which will obscure both kidneys, but primarily the right. Consequently, it is their feeling that ^{197}Hg Chlormerodrin will often fail to localize the kidneys in uremic patients, whereas radioactive chelates may be useful for these purposes. This authors recommend ^{99m}Tc DTPA for renal imaging studies in the presence of uremia, but recommend also ^{113m}In or ^{111}In DTPA. It is his feeling, on the basis of studies reviewing a large group of patients with BUN's above 65 mg-%, that rapid sequential and static imaging techniques, after injection of radiochelates, will result in useful renal images in about 75% of the cases. They do feel that visualization may depend upon when in the course of the illness the study is performed. If it is performed during the phase of ascending BUN in acute renal failure, the radionuclide chelates will usually demonstrate better intrarenal concentration and consequent kidney visualization than if the study is performed several days after the parenchymal insult. Later in the course of established renal failure they feel that there is a greater likelihood of better visualization if such a study is performed following hemodialysis.

In a study by BERNSTEIN et al. (1967), a dual radionuclide technique was used experimentally in dogs to evaluate tubular damage and recovery following experimentally induced ischemia obtained by clamping the renal artery for 90 min. By inducing two renograms, one obtained with ^{125}I-labeled diatrizoate, which is handled by glomerular filtration, and one with ^{131}I Hippuran, which is handled only 20% by filtration and 80% by tubular secretion, the normal tubular participation could be clearly seen. Following the 90 min of renal ischemia, the two curves became identical, indicative of tubular damage, and in time, they started to differ again as a signal of tubular recovery. Experimentally the same pattern could be produced by administration of Benemid, which blocks the tubular secretion of Hippuran. To our knowledge this has not been utilized clinically, but with the newer technetium-labeled chelates this should be a genuine possibility using the scintillation camera.

Several studies concerning the hemodynamics in acute renal failure have thrown a little more light upon the possible pathogenesis. HOLLENBERG et al. (1972), and later PEDERSEN and LADEFOGED (1973), demonstrated that the renal blood flow as well as intrarenal blood flow distribution was changed in acute renal failure. They demonstrated this by an external counting technique with ^{133}Xe and ^{131}I-labeled albumin. They found that the cortical blood flow was reduced to approximately one-fifth of the normal in the oliguric phase, and during this same phase, they found that the cortical fraction of the total blood flow was reduced to 66% against the normal of 92%. They further demonstrated that this blood flow reduction was due to a vascular resistance in the kidney which was about 4 times that of normal. They concluded that a reduced filtration pressure in the kidney, owing to an afferent arterial contraction, was the most likely explanation in the pathogenesis of acute renal failure. These findings probably explain why ^{131}I Hippuran imaging appears superior to the use of ^{99m}Tc DTPA, since at least acutely filtration appears suppressed considerably more than tubular secretion.

FREEMAN et al. (1969) studied 19 patients with BUN and plasma creatinine concentrations ranging from 62–146 and 3.5–7.2 mg-%, respectively. They found that intravenous urography and ^{197}Hg Chlormerodrin renal imaging were inadequate in these patients. The prolonged transit time which previously had been demonstrated for ^{131}I Hippuran makes it possible for the diseased kidney to concentrate the Hippuran even when the chlormerodrin concentration is not apparent. STAAB et al. (1973) used ^{131}I Hippuran for gamma scintillation images in 41 patients in acute or rapidly progressing chronic renal failure. They found that the ^{131}I Hippuran renal studies permitted correct prediction of eventual good renal function in 12 of 15 patients, with good visualization, and it predicted a poor outcome in 11 of 13 patients in whom the kidneys were not visualized. The serial renal radionuclide studies correctly predicted the ultimate outcome in 13 patients whose initial studies were indeterminate. They further found that information concerning kidney size, position, and presence of focal defects could be obtained during the oliguric phase. Even though renal failure with severe azotemia can be approached more readily today with the availability of hemodialysis, this is still a major undertaking in many places, and certainly the ability to be able to prognosticate concerning the outcome of acute renal failure is very important in the management of a patient.

One question is obviously how acute *is* acute; we have seen a patient with anuria for 3 months recover, and during this entire 3 months, visualization of the kidney could be obtained by ^{131}I-labeled Hippuran. Simultaneous attempts to obtain renal images with ^{99m}Tc DTPA were not as informative, although imaging could be obtained. It was the ability of the kidney to concentrate the Radiohippuran which made us feel that acute dialysis should be maintained, since recovery could not be excluded (Fig. 8). These studies were done on a patient who had a large hypernephroma of the lower pole of a solitary right kidney. The left kidney had been removed 6 years earlier due to hypernephroma. The dialysis team did not feel that chronic dialysis would be indicated in

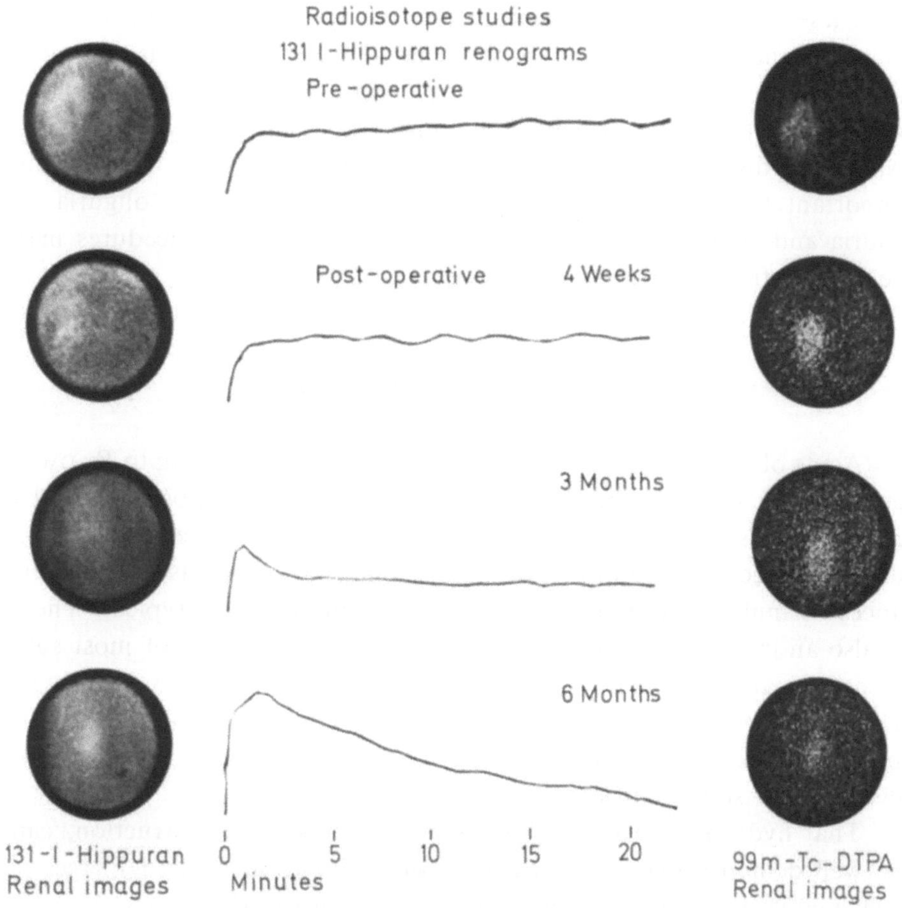

Fig. 8. Good visualization of kidney is seen throughout 3 months where patient was essentially anuric, indicative of recovery potential in acute tubular necrosis

a patient with recurrent neoplasm, and consequently a heminephrectomy with removal of the large hypernephroma was done, involving resection of the main renal vein which was filled with tumor. The upper pole, which was cooled during the surgical procedure, appeared viable, but as previously indicated, the patient was anuric 3 months following surgery. Only by pointing out the ability of this remaining right upper pole to concentrate Radiohippuran as indicated by the ability to obtain an image with a Gamma camera could we convince the dialysis team to continue the acute hemodialysis, and eventually the patient was able to recover enough renal function of this upper pole to discontinue hemodialysis.

These examples seem to demonstrate the usefulness of renal imaging in acute and occasionally chronic renal disease where it is desirable to obtain information concerning size, presence, and occasionally etiology without going to more invasive and considerably more risky procedures. As will be discussed under the section on hydronephrosis, it is equally important to rule out obstructive uropathy as a cause of oliguria or anuria and here again, the radionuclide renal imaging procedures may be very useful as a preliminary procedure.

F. Hydronephrosis

Acute obstruction of the renal outflow of urine, according to RADWIN et al. (1963), leads to changes that are very similar to those caused by renal artery stenosis, and a decrease in the rate of urine flow with a decrease in concentration of sodium and chloride as well as in the clearances of inulin, paraminohippurate, and Hippuran, are typical. There is also an increase in osmolality, and in the concentration of most substances apart from sodium and chloride, namely urea, inulin, PAH, Hippuran, and others. These changes occur at minimal elevation of pelvic pressure and are progressive. The decrease in inulin clearance may, however, appear somewhat later.

That hydronephrosis, i.e., either acute or chronic obstruction, can be well demonstrated by renography or scintillation camera images is well known and has been described by a number of authors. Equally important is the utilization of radionuclides for follow-up studies on patients where obstructive uropathy has been well demonstrated and where it is desirable to follow the course of events as well as the renal function without subjecting the patient to undue radiation and the possible risk of anaphylactic reaction to the injection of contrast media for intravenous urography. To the urologist it is also of importance to be able to distinguish between the patient who presents with back pain of unknown etiology, who may indeed have pain originating in the kidney or who may have completely unrelated pathology, be it back pain of muscular or skeletal etiology, or any number of causes unrelated to the urinary tract. Pain originating from obstructive uropathy involving dilatation of the renal pelvis or ureter or pain secondary to infections should be demonstrated by urinary tract infection and/or obstructive uropathy as can be well demonstrated in an early as well as delayed scintillation camera study.

In a patient with flank or back pain who has a negative urine and normal renal function with prompt appearance of radionuclides bilaterally and no indication of obstruction, it is most unlikely that such pain can be in any way connected with diseases of the urinary tract. In short, such pain can, in a very limited period of time with little or no discomfort or risk to the patient, be ruled within or out of the urinary tract system by rather simple procedures such as urinalysis and a scintillation camera study utilizing Radiohippuran.

The ability to predict the prognosis in terms of return of kidney function by radionuclides is perhaps worth commenting upon, and it should be understood that the utilization of radionuclides for this purpose is probably to expect more than there is any rational physiologic basis for. A kidney which has been obstructed for a period of time will unquestionably have a decrease in renal blood flow as well as filtration rate, and the utilization of radionuclides to predict the degree of recovery feasible by this maneuver alone cannot be expected, since neither the use of Radiohippuran, ^{133}Xe, or Hg-Chlormerodrin, regardless of the label of the mercury, can reveal any more than the present state of affairs concerning renal blood flow or filtration rate. In order to evaluate the possible prognosis, it is important to know the status of the contralateral kidney. If compensatory hypertrophy is present, it is unlikely that renal blood flow following release of obstruction will be any greater than what is presently demonstrated. In more acute situations, where compensatory hypertrophy has not occurred on the contralateral side, improvement in renal blood flow after release of obstruction may be feasible, but the radionuclide studies presently available will in no way predict the degree to which this may be possible.

In short, the utilization of radionuclides for the demonstration of obstructive uropathy is well recognized and with the scintillation camera, morphologic demonstrations and better clarification of obstruction is more feasible than with the old-fashioned renography; however, neither will demonstrate anything beyond the point of the present state of affairs at the time the study is being performed and no prognostication can be made unless the total kidney function, including the status of the contralateral kidney, is known.

It should be further added, as has been demonstrated also by JOEKES (1974), that the utilization of the gamma scintillation camera will allow evaluation of obstructive uropathy in portions of a kidney where renography would obviously not be able to distinguish, since no imaging here is feasible. As will be discussed later, many of the findings in urinary tract obstruction, i.e., a delayed peak and increasing accumulation over a prolonged period of time, are findings which are not necessarily specific and could in fact be found in acute tubular necrosis, decreased renal blood flow secondary to renal artery stenosis, or decreased cardiac output, as well as in rejection following kidney transplantation.

The utilization of renal imaging is exceedingly helpful in providing enough morphologic evidence which, together with follow-up studies, may be most helpful in a differential diagnosis as will be discussed later. It is thus important to remember that although the findings in urinary tract obstruction can be very dramatic, it is exceedingly important to combine such findings with other clinical parameters to make a specific diagnosis.

The other important aspect of the diagnosis of hydronephrosis involves the consideration of the volume of the collecting system and the quantitative evaluation of renal blood flow. In many instances, intravenous pyelography as well as radionuclide studies may reveal an obstructive pattern indicated by a dilated collecting system and accumulation of radionuclides or contrast media, depending upon the study performed. This may obviously indicate obstruction, but it may also indicate a dilated collecting system which may be congenital and constitute a system which imposes no danger to kidney function by virtue of any increased pressure. In order to appreciate the diagnostic problems, it is necessary to evaluate the specific influences upon renal blood flow.

Since the aim of the physician is obviously to preserve kidney function, it becomes questionable whether a dilated system, perhaps due to megaureter or congenital abnormalities involving some degree of caliectasis, is truly a pathologic condition requiring any therapeutic approach. It is important that the urologist treat the patient and not the x-ray, and this is one area where it is our feeling that the utilization of the ability to quantitate individual renal function can be most helpful acutely and as follow-up to evaluate the possible physiologic significance of a delayed drainage and a delayed peak from one or both kidneys.

In situations as illustrated here, where the radionuclide studies as well as intravenous urography indicated the presence of hydronephrosis, but where the kidney function was completely normal, we have followed a conservative approach, in order to see whether any decrease in kidney function occurred or whether the kidney function stayed normal. Any surgical approach to change an apparent obstructive pattern would be to improve and maintain kidney function. If kidney function is normal and is not deteriorating, it appears that therapy directed to change it would be in vain and at best result in no decrease in kidney function. Only if decreased renal blood flow or deterioration in renal blood flow is demonstrated does it seem that corrective measures are in order. The following cases will illustrate the point which we are trying to make.

The first patient was a 17-year-old female with a history of vague, right-sided back pain, but no history of urinary tract infections, no chills, fever, or hematuria. An intravenous pyelogram, shown in Fig. 9, was read as showing right hydronephrosis secondary to ureteropelvic junction obstruction. A retrograde pyelogram done elsewhere was said to confirm this, but upon questioning the patient, she volunteered that it caused some right-sided pain, but it was not, however, the same pain for which she originally sought medical attention.

A scintillation camera study was done and as seen in Fig. 10, the two kidneys appear alike, and quantitation indicated that 53% of her

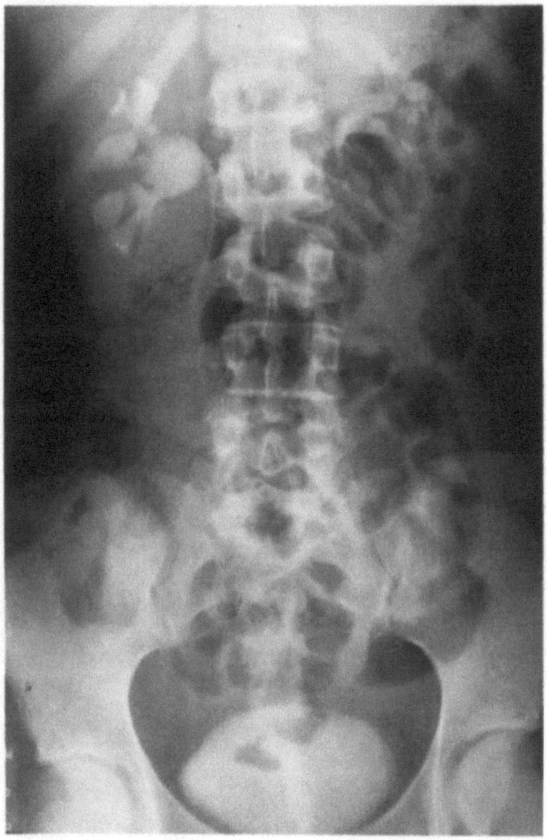

Fig. 9. Mild calicectasis and generous renal pelvis on right. Quantitation utilizing scintillation camera studies with ^{131}I Hippuran indicates normal renal blood flow bilaterally

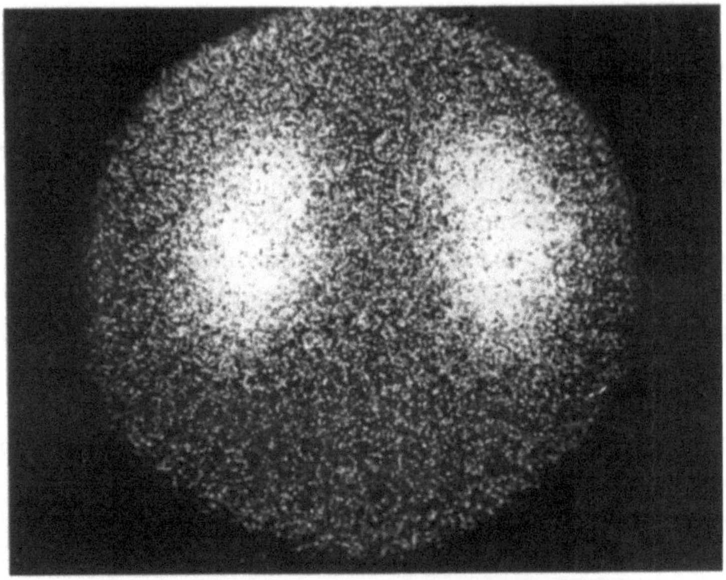

Fig. 10. Normal appearing uptake of Radiohippuran in both kidneys

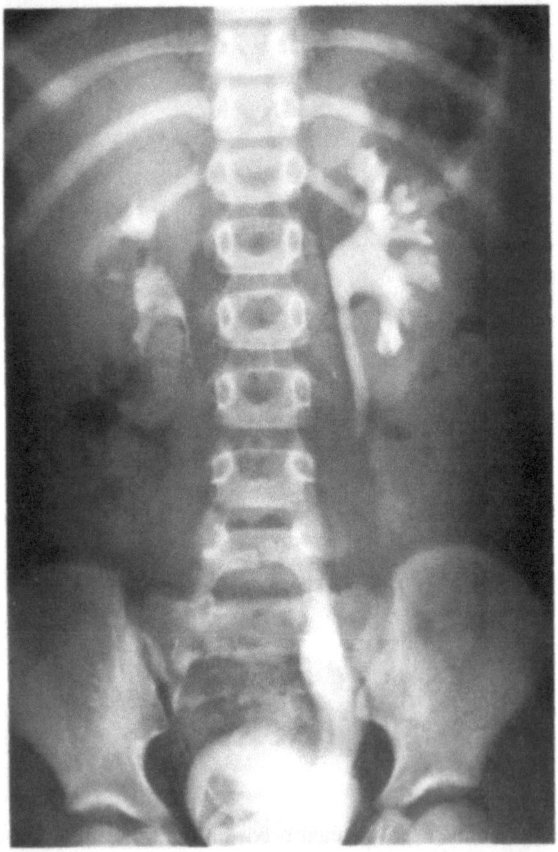

Fig. 11. Left-sided dilatation of collecting system as well as ureter, especially lower portion. Print-out of quantitation of Radiohippuran scintillation camera study is seen in Fig. 12

NAME L.M.

DATE 7-30-73

MATERIAL 131 I

SCINTILLATION CAMERA STUDY

TAPE # 18 PATIENT # 5170 SEX F AGE 5

BLOOD PRESSURE

PATIENT CONDITION Hydrated

TIME		R	%	L	%
0-1	COUNT	1792	51	1699	49
	CHANNEL	151	51	144	49
1-2		2477	49.4	2528	50.6
		176	48	179	52
2-3		2607	51	2488	49
		175	52	163	48
3-4		2131	49	2260	51
		153	49.8	154	50.2
4-5		1731	49	1836	51
		123	49.5	125	50.5
10		401	39	635	61
		40	40	60	60
15		0	0	10	
		0	0	1	
25		0	0	0	
		0	0	0	

MICROCURIES INJECTED 199

MICROCURIES EXCRETED IN 30 MINUTES

A) VOIDED 138 μci

B) RESIDUAL μci

C) TOTAL μci

URINE VOLUME 360 ML.

BLADDER COUNT IN MINUTES

BLADDER COUNT POST VOID

RESIDUAL URINE CALCULATED:

A) %

B) ML.

% OF RADIOHIPPURAN RETURNED IN 30 MIN.

A) VOIDED 70%

B) RESIDUAL

C) TOTAL

****

STUDY DIAGNOSIS:

NORMAL ☐

ABNORMAL R ☐ L ☐ B ☐

SPECIFIC

M.D.

Fig. 12. The 1–2 min uptake is practically identical with 50/50 distribution between two sides. Total return is normal, being 70%, and there is no great difference between excretory pattern on two sides. This constitutes a normal Radiohippuran study

total renal blood flow was present on the right. Her total function was within normal limits. She did have a slightly delayed peak on the right, but both kidneys were emptied in 25 min. This patient would likely have undergone a ureteropelvic junction repair, but on the basis of the renal scintillation camera studies, it is hard to see how her function could have been improved, and it is highly questionable if not very unlikely that her original right-sided pain had any connection with what we would consider a variation of normal. It is our routine to repeat such studies, to be sure that we are not dealing with a progressive situation, and if renal function is unchanged, we do not feel that this truly represents hydronephrosis.

Our next case is that of a 5-year-old female who presented with a urinary tract infection and nocturnal enuresis. An intravenous pyelogram indicated left ureterectasis, as shown in Fig. 11, and a camera study showed bilateral normal renal blood flow with equal distribution between the two kidneys (Fig. 12).

The patient was treated conservatively, and followed over several years; repeat scintillation camera studies 2 years later revealed no deterioration in function on either side. Again, it is our feeling that this type of functional evaluation can be helpful in deciding whether surgery has any place in the treatment of a given patient. It is obvious that this latter patient would not have benefited from surgery, since she had no deterioration in kidney function over a period of 2 years and, on antibacterial medication, no recurrence of urinary tract infection. It should be added that at no time was any reflux demonstrated by cystourethrography in this patient.

G. Renal Hypertension

Although patients with renovascular hypertension have been estimated to constitute only 6–8% of the total hypertensive population, the cures which have been feasible, by nephrectomy or vascular surgery, have been impressive enough to make it imperative that a proper diagnosis be made at an early time. The renogram as it was first developed has been used extensively as a noninvasive diagnostic tool to try to screen hypertensive patients who were potential candidates for corrective surgery. Again, the lack of ability to visualize portions of the kidney as well as the difficulty in accurate localization of the probes probably discouraged a number of investigators and clinicians in pursuing the utilization and development of the renogram technique.

The emergence of the gamma scintillation camera has led to a degree of sophistication which allows better quantitation with the capability of diagnosing segmental renal lesions, thus a more accurate screening of such patients. A number of publications have appeared on this subject, but it appears that all these studies employed renography without imaging, and thus without quantitation of uptake in designated areas of interest. These procedures are no longer considered to be sufficiently diagnostically accurate to apply to a situation where scintillation cameras are available. It further seems that such availability is highly desirable, not only in the area of diagnosis of renovascular disease, but also as has become apparent from this discussion, for many other urinary tract diseases.

WANG (1974), talks about "regional renograms" and compares to conventional renography, the "regional renograms" implying the utilization of the scintillation camera with information obtained from three different areas of each kidney. It was his feeling that there is a much better correlation between the regional renogram and the renal arteriogram than between the latter and the conventional renogram.

ROSENTHALL (1972), using the radionuclide approach to study renal disease in general and renovascular hypertension specifically, describes the Hg-chlormerodrin scan, radiopertechnetate perfusion, and serial 3 min-exposure ^{131}I Hippuran images, or serial 3-min ^{131}I Hippuran images followed by ^{99m}Tc glucoheptonate perfusion and static images. He subjected the radiotechnetium perfusion studies to data processing and used time activity histograms on playback for analysis on the transit through the kidneys and systemic circulation. The author concluded that this technique was considerably more sensitive than rapid sequence hypertensive intravenous pyelograms and more sensitive and informative than the conventional ^{131}I Hippuran renogram using paired external scintillation detectors.

FIGUEROA (1970) concluded that the perfection of the utilization of the renal scintigram has added much to aid the clinician in studying hypertensive renal disease, and KEANE and SCHLEGEL (1972) reported the use of the previously described screening procedure in the evaluation of possible renovascular disease in 424 patients. These scintillation camera studies, utilizing quantitation of radioactivity in the kidneys as well as in suspected segmental portions, if indicated, in conjunction with determination of total kidney function, revealed the possibility of renovascular disease in 56 of the 424 patients studied. Angiography was done in 35 of these 56 patients, of which 26 (74%) were found to have renovascular lesions. In comparing ^{131}I Hippuran renal scintillation camera studies, intravenous urography and angiography, no false-negative camera studies were found but a 12% incidence of false-negative intravenous urograms was described. A typical example of a segmental vascular lesion in the lower pole of the left kidney in a child with severe diastolic hypertension was demonstrated and as can be seen, renal histograms generated over upper and lower poles revealed the typical pattern of delayed uptake in the left lower pole (Fig. 13).

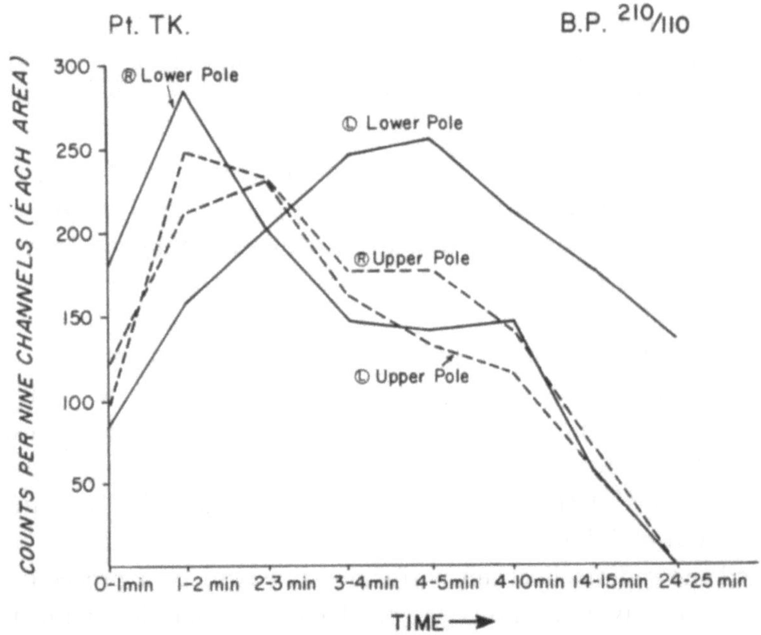

Fig. 13. Delayed peak and somewhat delayed excretion from left lower pole is contrasted with right lower pole as well as upper poles on right and left. These regional renal histograms were obtained by counting nine channels from right and left upper and lower poles respectively

Another example was that of a 51-year-old white female who had a long history of hypertension and urinary tract infections, and who in 1969 had a left nephrectomy for staghorn calculus. She was first referred here in 1970 for urologic evaluation because of azotemia and a blood pressure of 250/130. Intravenous pyelogram showed a solitary right kidney with hyperconcentration and delayed emptying of the upper pole (Fig. 14). The ^{131}I Hippuran rapid sequence scintillation camera study demonstrated delayed peaking and delayed emptying of the upper pole (Fig. 15). It was felt that this was compatible with duplication of the right renal artery and stenosis of the artery to the upper pole. This was confirmed by arteriography (Fig. 16) as well as at surgery during which saphenous vein aortorenal bypass graft was accomplished.

Postoperatively she underwent brisk diuresis with improvement of her azotemia and a scintillation camera study showed that the peak activity from the upper pole was now earlier than that from the lower pole (Fig. 17).

The possible discrepancy between renal physical mass and renal functioning mass as a parameter useful in determining relative renal ischemia

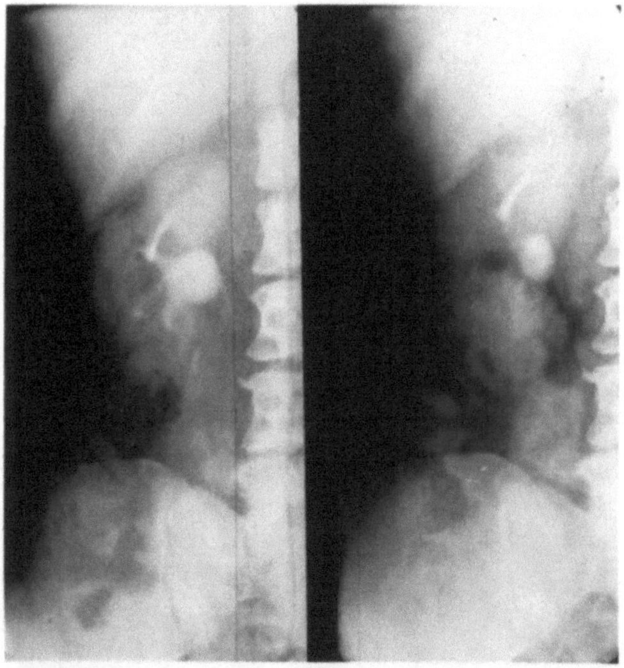

Fig. 14. Intravenous pyelogram on patient with solitary right kidney and severe diastolic hypertension. Pyelogram on left demonstrates filling of upper and lower calyces and some renal scarring is obvious. Pyelogram on right is taken at 15 min after injection and shows that lower pole has already emptied while contrast media is retained in upper pole and pelvis

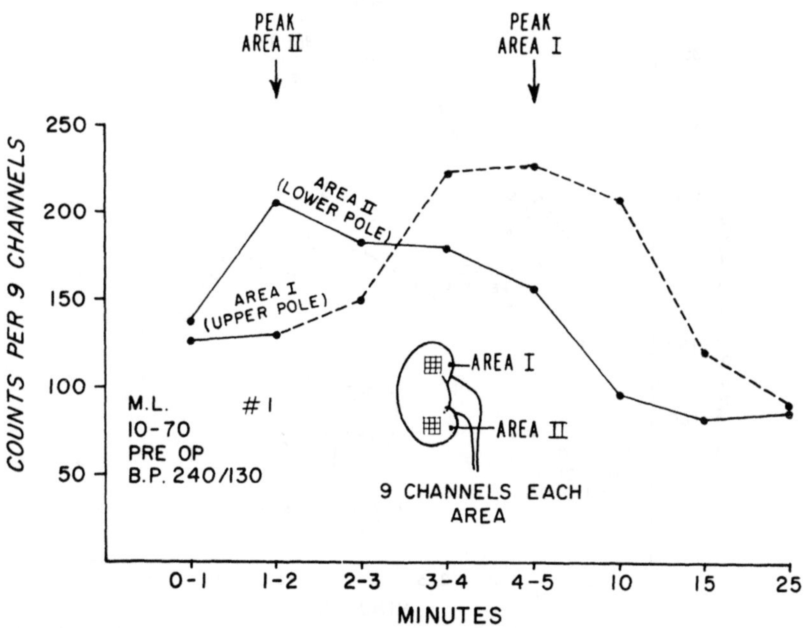

Fig. 15. Regional histograms generated over upper and lower pole of right kidney of patient whose intravenous pyelogram is depicted in Fig. 14. Upper pole which retained contrast medium longer shows typical delay in peak corresponding to finding seen in Fig. 16, demonstrating stenosis of artery supplying upper two-thirds of right kidney

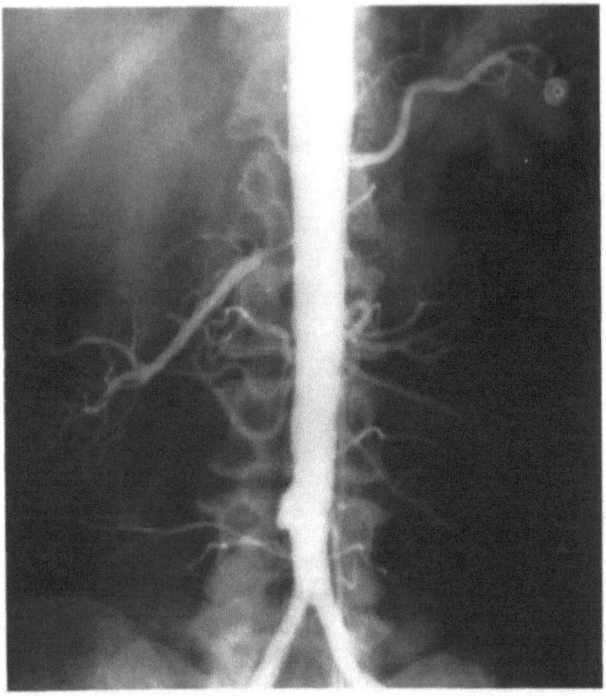

Fig. 16. Severe stricture is seen in most proximal take-off of renal artery supplying upper two-thirds of right kidney; lower pole is supplied by just a small branch coming off much further down the aorta

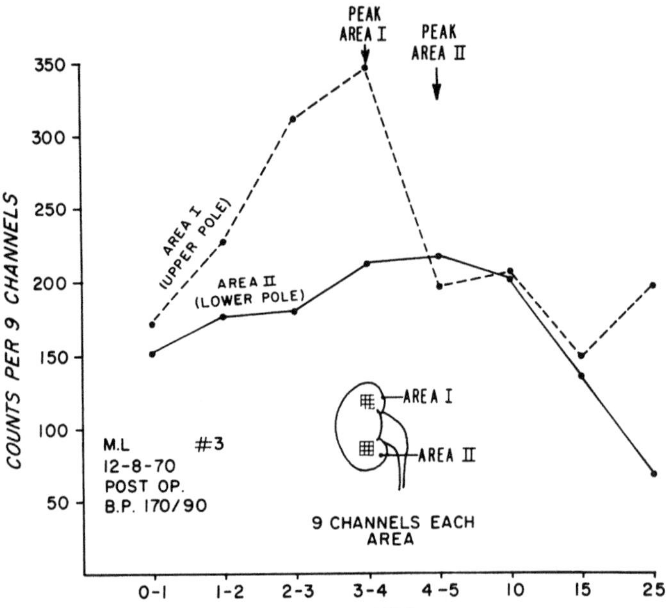

Fig. 17. Regional renal histograms on patient whose angiogram is seen in Fig. 16 following surgery, now demonstrating earlier peak from upper pole after revascularization has been done utilizing saphenous vein bypass

was proposed in 1967 by SCHLEGEL et al., based upon animal experimentation of studies done in 1961. Utilization was made of ^{203}Hg Neohydrin camera studies as a method for determining functioning renal mass and roentgenographic determination of renal area as a method for determining physical renal mass. In 20 patients operated upon for suspected unilateral renal hypertension, a disparity between these two parameters seemed to correlate well with the surgical outcome.

The problem of determination of renal mass, however, is more complicated than is apparent, as was well demonstrated by HODSON in 1961, in whose paper it was demonstrated that significant changes in renal size occur resulting from the lowering of blood pressure with Pentothal anesthesia. Calculated in renal volume, he reports as much as a 40% decrease. What was even more striking was the difference in the renal volume decrease in patients with unilateral ischemic renal disease secondary to renal artery stenosis. In such an instance, normal kidneys shrank about 42% in volume, while the ischemic kidneys shrank only 25% in volume due to lowering of the blood pressure. Since in such patients a lowering of the blood pressure to normotensive levels could equalize the size of the two kidneys, where in the state of hypertension the ischemic kidney would be smaller than its normal mate, it becomes increasingly obvious that determination of renal mass is not such a simple matter, since it is necessary to define the condition under which renal area or mass is determined. It appears that not only may ischemic kidneys shrink less than a nonischemic kidney when the blood pressure is lowered, but it may shrink even more if the blood pressure is lowered below a critical level, at which autoregulation is no longer feasible. If a significant unilateral renal artery lesion is present, a normal perfusion pressure and blood flow of such a kidney may only be possible by elevation of systemic blood pressure. Lowering such blood pressure may create a decrease in perfusion pressure on the affected side, so that the lowering of the blood pressure to normotensive levels may seriously change the blood flow or perfusion pressure in the kidney with the stenotic renal artery, since autoregulation ceases when the arterial mean blood pressure drops below 90 mm Hg.

Utilizing ^{203}Hg Neohydrin, SCHLEGEL et al. (1971) demonstrated the use of scintillation camera studies in evaluation of renal volume resulting from the administration of vasoactive drugs. SEMPREBENE et al. (1972), utilizing Radiohippuran renography and split function renal tests, concluded that neither of these determinations under basal conditions were reliable indices of the anatomic status of the contralateral kidney while their modifications during infusion of trimethaphan camphorsulfonate (Arfonad) provided a more accurate means of predicting surgical results. They found that when a delay of transit time appeared on the renogram and the renal plasma flow decreased in the contralateral kidney during Arfonad administration, constructive procedures were advisable, while nephrectomy, according to these authors, should never be done, since it would fail to correct hypertension. They further concluded that when a delay of transit time was observed under basal conditions, positive results could be obtained only by contralateral nephrectomy after revascularization of the kidney with main arterial disease.

It has been our practice in screening hypertensive patients to obtain first an ^{131}I Hippuran study as described previously with the patient in a well-hydrated state, and off antihypertensive therapy. The same study is then repeated with the patient's blood pressure lowered to normotensive levels and this will frequently exaggerate the findings that already were suggested by the original study, i.e., an increase in transit time with a considerable delay in peak of the uptake of radionuclide and considerable delay in excretion.

We have previously attempted to use Arfonad; however, the inconsistency with which we were able to lower the blood pressure made it of somewhat doubtful value, and we are presently using diazoxide (Hyperstat) and this seems to give rather promising results.

We rarely use anything but ^{131}I Hippuran in screening for a possible renal artery lesion in hypertensive patients, since the results obtained here appear to be much more informative than those obtained with Technetium-labeled chelates. If on the scintiphoto an unequal distribution of the Radiohippuran appears evident, electronic flagging of various areas of the kidney is done, and a renal histogram is generated to show possible differences in blood flow, transit time, as well as emptying for the purpose of demonstrating segmental lesions. Such studies can also be done in suspected cases in an oblique position, demonstrating differences between anterior and posterior portions of the kidney, a finding which may be as common if not indeed more common than differences involving upper, lower, and middle portions as detected in the AP view.

In evaluating hypertensive patients and in attempting to prognosticate as to the outcome of surgical procedures, we have found it to be of paramount importance to have an accurate determination of the total kidney function, i.e., the actual renal blood flow on the contralateral side, since a decrease in total function is usually indicative of disease in the contralateral kidney which often makes treatment by nephrectomy of doubtful value. Overall, it appears to us that attempted surgical correction of a unilateral renovascular lesion rarely results in a cure if the contralateral kidney is not normal, i.e., has not undergone compensatory hypertrophy. If, however, the total kidney function is normal, equally good results can be expected from either renal artery repair or nephrectomy.

If bilateral renal arterial stenosis exists, the situation is somewhat more complicated, since this may explain a decrease in total renal function and then yet, surgical intervention may be curative. Usually such a situation is present with one kidney being much more severely affected than the other. Consequently, the end results as far as scintillation camera studies are concerned will be the typical demonstration of possible renal artery stenosis on one side with a delayed peak and delayed excretion and possibly decreased renal blood flow on one side with a contralateral kidney which has not undergone compensatory hypertrophy and for all practical purposes can represent parenchymal renal disease or renal artery stenosis to a minor extent. Only by combining the evaluation with total as well as split renal vein renin determinations and renal angiography can an assessment be made. Evaluation of urinary osmolality may also be helpful in deciding the possible prognosis.

In such a situation, a nephrectomy of the most severely involved kidney will often result in an aggravation of hypertension while repair of the renal artery may be curative and in some instances, bilateral renal artery revascularization may be needed.

Although the significant scintillation camera studies in unilateral renal artery disease causing hypertension are quite typical, showing an increased transit time with delayed peak and a delayed excretory phase, such findings can occur in other situations such as chronic pyelonephritis, partial obstruction, rejection, and acute tubular necrosis. This problem, however, is not as serious as it may sound, since hypertension does not always accompany the latter pathologic states, and the problem would primarily arise in situations where bilateral renal artery disease of the main renal arteries were present. Most of the other conditions referred to, if bilateral, would result in a decrease in total kidney function. As reported in the paper by KEANE and SCHLEGEL (1972), as previously described, there were no false-negative camera studies while there were 7 patients out of 35 with a false-positive camera study (26%). It is our hope that evaluation utilizing the same scintillation camera technique with lowering of the blood pressure will decrease the number of false-positive camera studies, but further work must be done along these lines.

H. Renal Transplantation

Acute tubular necrosis, ureteral, or pelvic obstruction, as well as renal artery stenosis, are pathologic entities which can occur as a result of renal transplantation. The additional factor responsible for oliguria or anuria in the transplant patient is that of rejection. The use of radionuclides for monitoring the function of the grafted kidney has become more and more an integral part of renal transplantation. The actual physiologic result of rejection has been studied intensively by numerous investigators utilizing ^{133}Xe, Neohydrin, and Radiohippuran. ROSEN et al. (1968) demonstrated that as rejection progressed in a homotransplanted kidney in the dog, xenon studies and radioautography indicated that this correlated with a decrease in the volume of cortex perfused by Component I. Similar studies in man indicate that Component I of the xenon curve perfuses the renal cortex in man, and it was noted that urine formation ceased in three subjects at a time when some renal blood flow continued to be supplied to Component I at a normal flow rate and normal systemic blood pressure. These data seem to indicate that certain parts of the cortex can be perfused normally without production of urine, and it is suggested that the anuria could be due to failure of filtration resulting from localized areas of low perfusion pressure in the kidney or excessive reabsorption.

RETIK et al. (1969) showed in renal allographs in dogs treated with immunosuppressive drugs that cortical ischemia occurred early in rejection before there was any histologic evidence of vascular lesions. They further mentioned that the rapid reversibility of cortical ischemia with reversal of rejection indicates that active vasoconstriction could play an important role in the ischemia and pathogenesis of renal allograph rejection.

Further use of ^{133}Xe has been reported by LEWIS et al. (1967) who measured renal blood flow at the time of operation. They found in 13 living donor transplants, flow in the recipient after reestablishment of the vascular supply was essentially the same as in the donor 43 min earlier, and had a tendency to increase. In all of these instances, urine output started immediately. In cadaver transplants, they found that the average initial flow value in the recipient was lower than in the living donor group and had a tendency to decline. In this group, only two out of ten kidneys produced urine immediately. They summarize by stating that the measurement of renal blood flow at the time of kidney transplantation is an important check on kidney function, and they feel that values below 100 ml/min/100 g of renal tissue are not compatible with eventual renal function. An additional use of ^{133}Xe was reported by CHO et al. in 1974. They evaluated the potential function of kidneys harvested from a cadaver by determining renal blood flow using ^{133}Xe with the kidney maintained on the pump. They feel that the method is of potential importance in the evaluation of cadaver kidneys of marginal quality.

In 1965, MOBLEY and SCHLEGEL reported on the accumulation in the transplanted kidney of Radiohippuran as a signal of rejection, a publication which was shortly followed by similar observations by FIGUEROA et al. (1968), an observation which to this day appears to be the prototype of a phenomenon which is presently studied more frequently utilizing the scintillation camera than renography or renal scan as was used in the past. A variant of this phenomenon, mainly the utilization of the bladder to kidney ratio of radioactivity following injection of ^{131}I Hippuran was published by HAYES in 1971, who stated that a decrease in this ratio seems to be one of the earliest and most sensitive indicators of acute allograph rejection. Several other publications have attested to the usefulness of radionuclide evaluation in the transplanted patient as a simple, noninvasive procedure which often will signal problems before clinical symptomatology or changes in clearances will alert the physician, and thus be helpful in initiating earlier corrective measures.

In 1974, SALVATIERRO et al. reported the use of renal scintiphotography with ^{131}I Hippurate in evaluating renal failure and complications in more than 500 transplant patients. They state that this diagnostic test has become their principle method of evaluation and follow-up of renal transplants, particularly in the early posttransplant period. They feel that this approach will allow the physician to accurately distinguish tubular necrosis, rejection, and other complications in the early posttransplant period. They further state that the approach is one of simplicity, safety, and accuracy, which makes it of great value to the transplant surgeon and their patients. These investigators also did direct scintiphotography of blood flow distribution in the grafts with ^{99m}Tc DTPA, which they primarily used as a supplemental examination in selected instances of suspected vascular compromise. These investigators point out a very important part of the handling of the posttransplant patient, which will ease the known difficulties in distinguishing between entities which using simple renography are practically indistinguishable, i.e., the distinction between rejection, acute tubular necrosis, obstruction to outflow, and renal artery obstruction. This important point which is crucial is that a baseline Radiohippuran scintiphotographic study be obtained on the first postoperative day, and they also point out that the control or first scintiphotographic study should not be done until 24 h after transplantation, because renal damage produced by anoxia will usually reach its maximum at the 24-h point. It is their feeling that further renal deterioration as a result of tubular necrosis is not seen after this period, and if further deterioration in the scintiphotographic studies does occur, after 24 h, it is usually due to rejection.

It is the opinion of these authors that the ^{99m}Tc radiopharmaceuticals are of little value, while the ^{131}I Hippuran is the radiopharmaceutical of choice at the present time. The authors further point out that there are two particular problems in which scintiphotography is of limited value, namely in the hypertensive patient with suspected renal artery stenosis in the transplant graft and the patient with a mild ureteral obstruction. One final complication of renal transplant not mentioned previously is that of ureteral urinary extravasation, which can be well demonstrated by scintillation camera studies utilizing ^{131}I Hippuran (Fig. 18).

Not everyone agrees that the ^{99m}Tc radiopharmaceuticals are of little value in evaluating patients with kidney transplants; ZUM WINKEL et

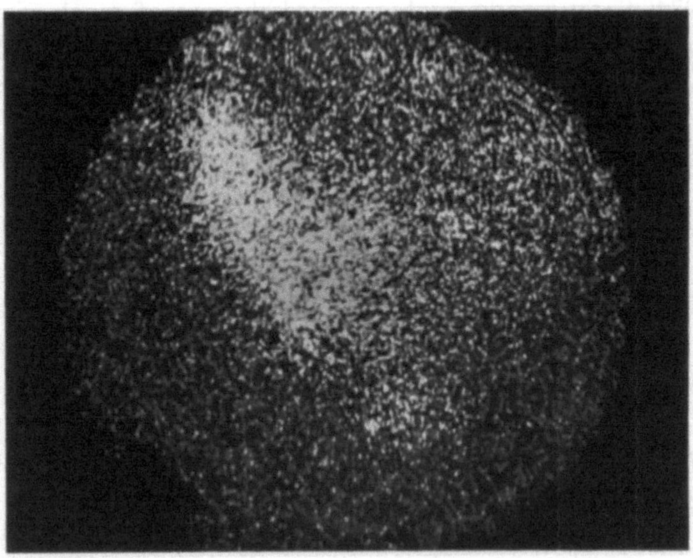

Fig. 18. Radiohippuran uptake in renal transplant is clearly seen but the whole right aspect of the scintiphoto shows diffuse radiation indicative of urinary extravasation. Bladder can faintly be seen in lowermost portion of picture

al. (1972), feel that a bolus injection of such radiopharmaceuticals are of the greatest value in establishing the patency of the new reanastomosed vascular pathway. ROSENTHALL et al. (1974) also pointed to the importance of sequential radionuclide studies in the diagnosis of acute tubular necrosis and rejection and stated that isolated studies can be misleading, since it is the change in function that is crucial to an early and accurate diagnosis. It is their feeling that the Radiohippurate renal uptake determinations and the Radiopertechnetate renograms can anticipate the biochemical and clinical impressions of rejection by as much as 48 h, and they feel that the utilization of these techniques assume an even greater importance while patients are on dialysis when biochemical determinations are almost meaningless. They suggest that the possible use of ^{131}I fibrinogen will separate the two entities, since fibrin is deposited in the kidney in rejection but not in acute necrosis.

The occasional dilatation of the calyceal system and/or ureter in the transplant patient sometimes on intravenous urography suggests obstructive uropathy and the question of surgical intervention becomes important. If indeed obstruction exists, it is obviously a situation which should be corrected, but as discussed under the section on obstructive uropathy, the utilization of radionuclides incorporating quantitation and determination of renal function can be helpful in assessing such a situation. It is not uncommon to find dilatation of the collecting system which may be secondary to some partial rejection of the ureter without any anatomical obstruction. We have seen patients who showed no deterioration in kidney function over several years, yet the radiologic appearance was that of hydronephrosis and certainly suggestive of obstructive uropathy (Figs. 19, 20).

The accumulation and delay in excretion of radiopaque media or radionuclides may be of little significance if it does not result in any deterioration of kidney function and thus indicates that no back pressure or renal damage has occurred. Our primary purpose in dealing with transplant patients, or for that matter, any patient with urinary tract abnormalities, is to preserve kidney function, and if it appears unlikely that an improvement in kidney function will result from surgery and that in fact no deterioration in function has resulted from the apparent obstructive uropathy, then clearly surgery for relief of a suggested anatomical obstruction is not the proper approach.

The utilization of the quantitative Radiohippuran scintillation camera study, incorporating determination of residual urine, if any, and return of the injected dose in 30 min, has been applied by us for many years

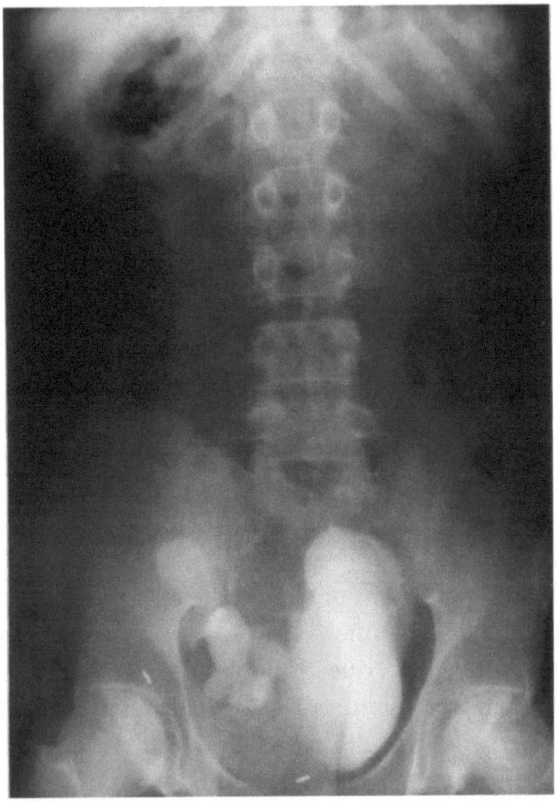

Fig. 19. Intravenous pyelogram of transplanted kidney showing great deal of calicectasis with bladder visualizing next to kidney

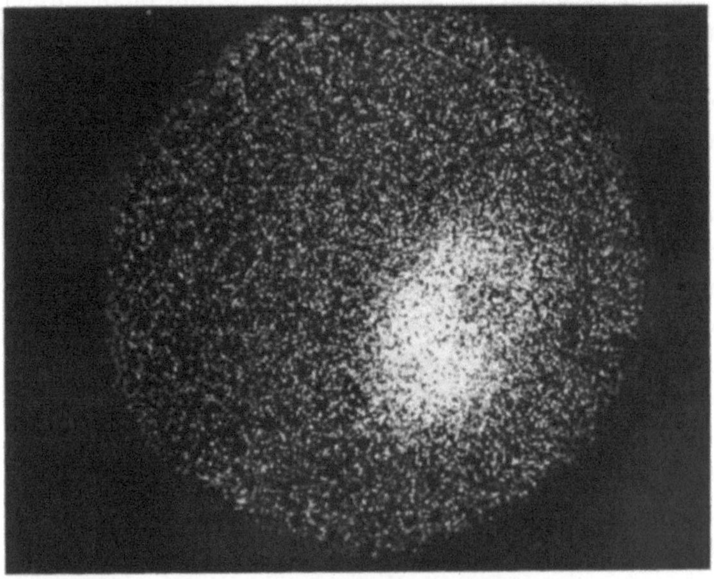

Fig. 20. Scintiphoto of transplant of which intravenous pyelogram is depicted in Fig. 19. Orientation here is reversed, but it demonstrates good uptake in 0–3 min exposure

to potential transplant donors as a first step. If this study is abnormal, either in terms of decreased kidney function or in terms of unilateral abnormality, such information combined with urinalysis may in a matter of 30 min make further evaluation unnecessary, at least as far as the potential status as a donor is concerned. We have experienced many times that the 30 min return of injected Radiohippuran is a more reproducible and better index of kidney function than repeated 24-h creatinine clearances and certainly less bothersome and less time consuming. If unilateral renal pathology exists, this may not necessarily be detected by intravenous urography and the quantitative evaluation of individual kidney function in this situation is of crucial importance for donor and recipient alike.

J. Radionuclides in the Pediatric Patient

Determination of clearances by the classical standard technique, as has previously been discussed, is not useful in a clinical setting, and if this statement is correct in adults, it is even more so in children. DONATH (1971) compared in a large number of children the standard clearance techniques with single injection radionuclide procedures in determination of glomerular filtration rate and effective renal plasma flow. The author concludes that although the correctness of the radionuclide procedure using a single injection has never been proven, the method gives sufficient precise results in practice and are recommended because of the technical simplicity for patient as well as for the laboratory technician. Similar studies were done by VOGELI et al. (1971) who feel that the indications for the use of single injection technique in pediatric patients are: (1) the patient with oliguria, a "Bricker bladder," ureterosigmoidostomy, as well as in patients with hydronephrosis or vesicoureteral reflux; and (2) patients with a greater than average risk of urinary tract infection by catheterization.

Although the radiation exposure is minimal with the above mentioned techniques, the use of renography and in particular, scintillation camera studies where somewhat higher dosages are required, have led to studies of radiation dosimetry for various radionuclides in children. HENK et al. in 1967 studied 30 patients by whole body counting and thyroid uptake measurements following routine ^{131}I Hippuran renography and calculated the radiation dose to kidneys, thyroid, bladder wall, and gonads.

It was found that most of the activity retained was in the thyroid gland, primarily resulting from free iodide in the injected material. The thyroid dose was found to be on the order of 1 rem and this could be reduced by a factor of 7–10 by blocking the thyroid or using iodide-free Hippuran. The gonadal dose was found to be less than 2 millirems, which is about 1% of the dose resulting from an intravenous urogram. These authors concluded that renography constituted a negligible radiation hazard to the patient. CONWAY, in 1972, reported on experiences from the Children's Memorial Hospital in Chicago, Illinois, and in his review, the reader can find recommendations for a dose schedule with various radionuclides. CONWAY points out that radiation to an infant is greater for a given amount of radiopharmaceutical than to an older child or adult, and that this is particularly important when using ^{131}Iodine in the newborn. The thyroid has a great affinity for iodine in the first few weeks of life, and he consequently recommends that such studies be postponed for at least 2–3 weeks following birth unless the diagnosis is of paramount importance. It is their routine to give all pediatric patients who receive ^{131}iodine Lugol's solution prior to and for 5 days following the examination, unless the patient has proven allergy to iodine or normal renal function. If the kidney function is normal, they still give Lugol's solution prior to the radionuclide study but omit it thereafter. This article also contains valuable suggestions for the immobilization of the pediatric patient, which is particularly important with infants and children between 6 months and 3 years of age. CONWAY points out in his review the advantages of obtaining initial images with the detector beneath the child to decrease the apprehension since suspending the massive-appearing detector above him may further increase the anxiety already present. The usual procedure at Children's Memorial Hospital is to administer all medications, such as Lugol's solution or potassium perchlorate, upon arrival and then inject the radionuclide before the sedation has taken full effect. We prefer to insert a scalp vein needle with its plastic connector so that the actual injection of the radionuclide can take place without the commotion associated with insertion of the needle, and so that true zero time of the injection of the radionuclide can be done with the child properly relaxed. Further work in regard to radiopharmaceutical dosimetry in pediatrics was published by KEREIAKES et al. (1972), and contains information on the various parameters involved in radiopharmaceutical dosimetry in pediatrics, incorporating age groups from newborns to age 15.

RADWIN and NOVOSELSKY published in 1967 a paper describing the potential usefulness of the gamma scintillation camera in pediatric urologic diagnosis. They pointed out that studies using Hippuran labeled with ^{131}iodine have shown that the kidney with even mild chronic pyelonephritis does not excrete small volumes as well as does the normal kidney, although the handling of a large volume may be similar. They demonstrated this by performing sequential camera studies under conditions of water diuresis and comparing them to those done with Pitressin-induced antidiuresis. These studies indicated that under conditions of water diuresis the radionuclide is excreted equally from the two kidneys, but under the condition of antidiuresis, there is hold-up on the diseased side.

BUESCHEN et al. (1974), using the method of SCHLEGEL et al. (1970), studied the usefulness of the renal scintillation camera study in 443 children. The camera studies and an intravenous urogram were reviewed in 271 patients. They concluded that the test provided information about the total renal function and relative function of both kidneys by a noninvasive technique which required only 30 min. They also pointed out that no surgically significant pathology was missed by the radionuclide study with the gamma camera, provided that quantitative analysis was done.

O'NEILL and MAXFIELD (1972), utilizing the gamma scintillation camera and ^{131}I Hippuran in 23 newborn infants, found that the camera renogram proved to be more reliable in terms of quality of the study than intravenous urography. They further indicated in their findings that the renogram demonstrated findings in at least three instances not demonstrated by the infusion pyelogram, and further emphasized that the camera renogram involves less radiation than the pyelogram. It is their suggestion that the camera renogram deserves further evaluation as a screening tool to be used in those neonates in whom such studies are indicated.

It thus appears that there is general agreement that the use of radionuclides in diagnostic pediatric urology has a great deal to offer, not only in terms of diagnostic accuracy, but also in terms of a lower radiation dose to the body in general and specifically the gonads than that which is achieved by radiology, perhaps apart from the thyroid which can be adequately blocked by prior administration of Lugol's solution. The utilization of radionuclides in the diagnosis of reflux will be discussed under the section dealing with the bladder.

K. Radionuclides in Bladder Pathology Including Vesicoureteral Reflux

STRAUSS and BLAUFOX in 1970, and SCHLEGEL and BAKULE in the same year, published a technique for calculating residual urine without urethral catheterization utilizing radionuclides. STRAUSS and BLAUFOX (1970) incorporated a study of 30 patients, 20 of them with obstructive uropathy who were evaluated with renography by injection of 25 μCi of ^{131}I Hippuran. Approximately 45 min after injection, they estimated the radioactivity detected in the bladder area after the patient had urinated, and found that their calculation of mean residual volume compared exceedingly well with the determinations made by catheterization. They also used this method to determine urine flow rates in patients and felt that this method was accurate and reliable and recommended that it be used in preference to urethral catheterization to determine residual urine volume and urine flow rates in patients with lower urinary tract obstruction. A similar approach to the determination of residual urine was reported by SCHLEGEL and BAKULE in 1970, as a part of the screening test utilizing the gamma scintillation camera in a state of adequate hydration and as part of the overall evaluation of the urinary tract. This approach not only will determine the residual urine accurately, if the kidneys are empty at approximately 30 min after the injection, but will also allow calculation of total kidney function even if some residual urine is present.

A paper by HARBERT et al. in 1970 points out that a full bladder can produce a renogram pattern of prolonged transit time which may interfere with the proper diagnosis and they consequently recommend that patients void before each renogram since bladder distention may produce an abnormal pattern. We have in the routine screening procedures which have been described previously, purposely not asked the patient to urinate before the scintillation camera study since this may interfere with an adequate determination of residual urine. It is our feeling that the total return is not greatly influenced by the bladder filling unless it is excessive and that the excretory phase of the renal histogram is not terribly important unless it is different on the two sides. We find it exceedingly rare that the kidneys are not empty in 30 min in any well-hydrated patient who has a normal urinary tract, and if the patient urinates before the camera study, emptying may in some individuals be difficult if insufficient volumes of urine are present in the bladder. If any question should arise in terms of abnormalities, a repeat study can always be performed with the patient emptying the bladder prior to the study.

Vesicoureteral Reflux

Vesicoureteral reflux is a situation which seems to invoke almost a passionate and dogmatic approach on behalf of many urologists. Unfortunately the approach differs, but it appears that one thing can be agreed upon by everybody, namely the purpose of evaluation and treatment, which obviously is to preserve kidney function. Although vesicoureteral reflux is not limited to the pediatric patient, it is unquestionably more predominant and of greater concern in the child, and most commonly in the female child with recurrent urinary tract infections. Many approaches and recommendations have been made over the years, and several publications involving the use of radionuclides have appeared. Apart from the treatment of any acute urinary tract infection, the first study we routinely do is a gamma scintillation camera study utilizing ^{131}I-labeled Hippuran. It is the experience of the author that if the result of this is normal, meaning that there is identical renal blood flow bilaterally and a normal total renal blood flow, nothing further can be learned by an intravenous urogram unless there is evidence of segmental decrease in blood flow indicative of a duplicated system on one or both sides. Our next step is a cystogram to detect the presence or absence of vesicoureteral reflux, and if such is present in the face of normal kidney function, conservative therapy with long-term antibacterial agents is our usual approach with frequent follow-up, i.e., every 6 months, utilizing quantitative evaluation of individual kidney function. If no recurrent infections occur and total as well as individual renal function remains unchanged and normal, suppressive antibacterial therapy is continued unless disappearance of vesicoureteral reflux is demonstrated, in which case antibacterial therapy is withdrawn (Evans et al., 1974).

A typical example is illustrated by a 7-year-old female who was originally seen 5 years ago with recurrent urinary tract infections. A gamma scintillation camera study showed normal kidney function and equal distribution between the two kidneys. An intravenous pyelogram was completely normal, and a voiding cystourethrogram (Fig. 21) showed bilateral reflux most pronounced on the right. The scintiphoto obtained

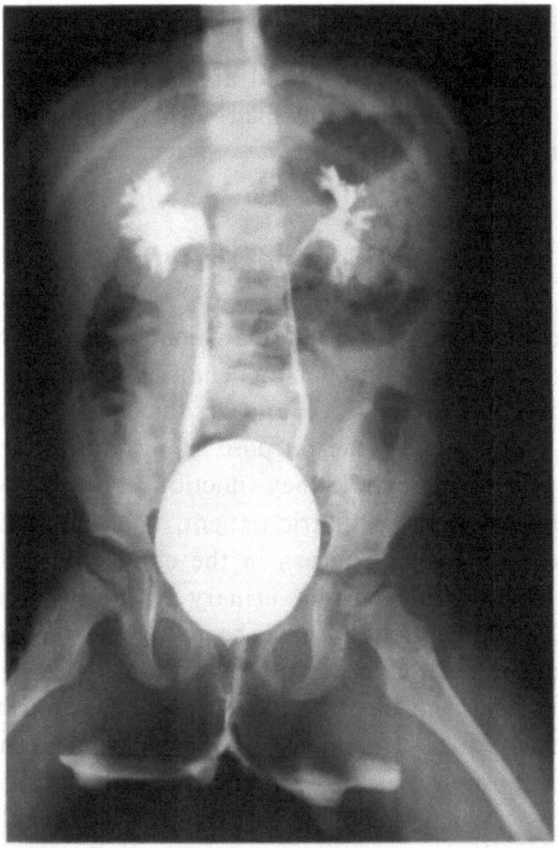

Fig. 21. Voiding cystourethrogram on female child showing gross bilateral reflux most pronounced on right

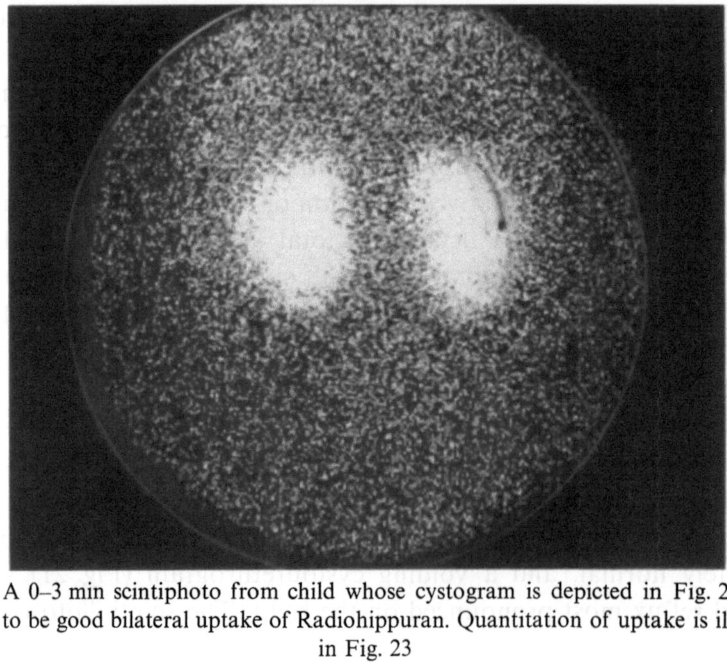

Fig. 22. A 0–3 min scintiphoto from child whose cystogram is depicted in Fig. 21. There appears to be good bilateral uptake of Radiohippuran. Quantitation of uptake is illustrated in Fig. 23

NAME C.K.

DATE 5/ 23/ 74

MATERIAL 131 I

SCINTILLATION CAMERA STUDY

TAPE # ? PATIENT # 2941 SEX w/f AGE 6yrs.

BLOOD PRESSURE 115/60

PATIENT CONDITION

hydrated well , had pt empty bladder before study

TIME	R	%	L	%
0-1 COUNT	2371	51	2357	49
CHANNEL	165	49	169	51
1-2	3575	51	3526	49
	194	51	184	51
2-3	4257	52	3971	48
	195	53	170	47
3-4	4455	55	3679	45
	168	51	161	49
4-5	4680	64	2680	36
	172	55	138	45
10	2685	81	625	19
	103	67	50	33
15	2006	92	186	8
	89	82	19	18
25	145	100	0	0
	15	100	0	0

MICROCURIES INJECTED 209

MICROCURIES EXCRETED IN 30 MINUTES

A) VOIDED 156 μci

B) RESIDUAL 0 μci

C) TOTAL 156 μci

URINE VOLUME 68 ML.

BLADDER COUNT IN 28 MINUTES 8159

BLADDER COUNT POST VOID 29

RESIDUAL URINE CALCULATED:

A) .3 %

B) 0 ML.

% OF RADIOHIPPURAN RETURNED IN 30 MIN.

A) VOIDED 75%

B) RESIDUAL 0

C) TOTAL 75%

****

STUDY DIAGNOSIS:

NORMAL ☐

ABNORMAL R ☐ L ☐ B ☐

SPECIFIC

M.D.

Fig. 23. Five years following detection of bilateral reflux in this now 6-year-old child, total kidney function is completely normal, being 75%, and distribution of renal blood flow between two kidneys is 51% and 49%, respectively. This pattern did not change over 5 years patient was followed, and reflux now has spontaneously disappeared

from the 0–3-min accumulation is shown in Fig. 22. The patient was followed conservatively over a 5-year period with repeat scintillation camera studies and repeat yearly cystograms which revealed disappearance of reflux on the left after 2–3 years and finally, disappearance of the reflux on the right at the end of 5 years. Figure 23 is a print-out of the quantitative scintillation camera study at the time bilateral reflux had ceased, and it illustrates that the 1–2 min uptake indicative of relative renal blood flow was equal with a perfectly normal renal function showing a return of the injected radionuclide of 75%.

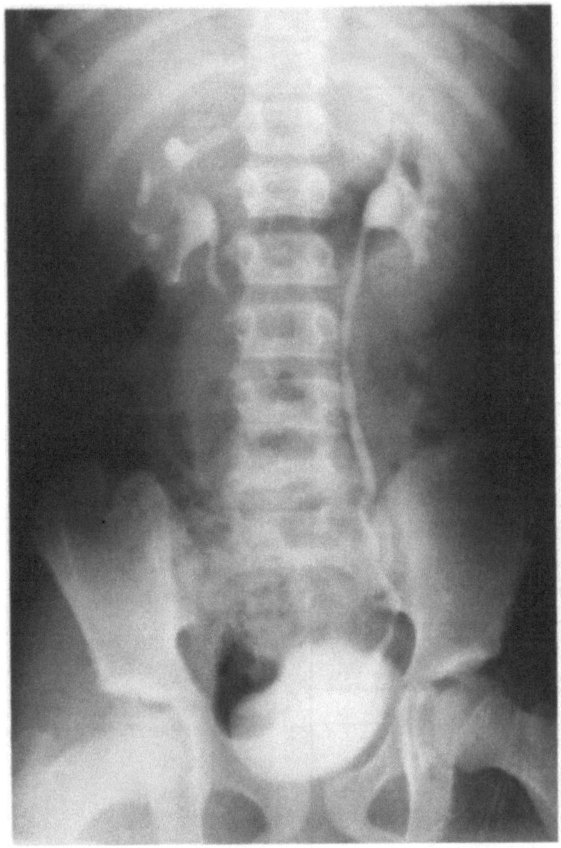

Fig. 24. Intravenous pyelogram on 10-year-old female with recurrent urinary tract infection. Right kidney shows blunting of calyces and thinning of cortex

In situations where individual or total kidney function is below normal, intravenous urography is naturally performed to evaluate the morphology in addition to cystourethrograms. If very little kidney function exists on one side as a result of recurrent urinary tract infection and compensatory hypertrophy is present in the contralateral kidney, sometimes unilateral nephrectomy may be in order.

Figure 24 shows an intravenous pyelogram on a 10-year-old female who presented at age 9 with recurrent urinary tract infection. It is apparent from the intravenous urogram that the right kidney is abnormal, and shows the results of chronic infection. Figure 25 is a renal scintiphoto with ^{131}I Hippuran showing poor function on the right, and Fig. 26 shows on the print-out of the quantitative studies that only 16% of the total and otherwise normal renal function is present on the right.

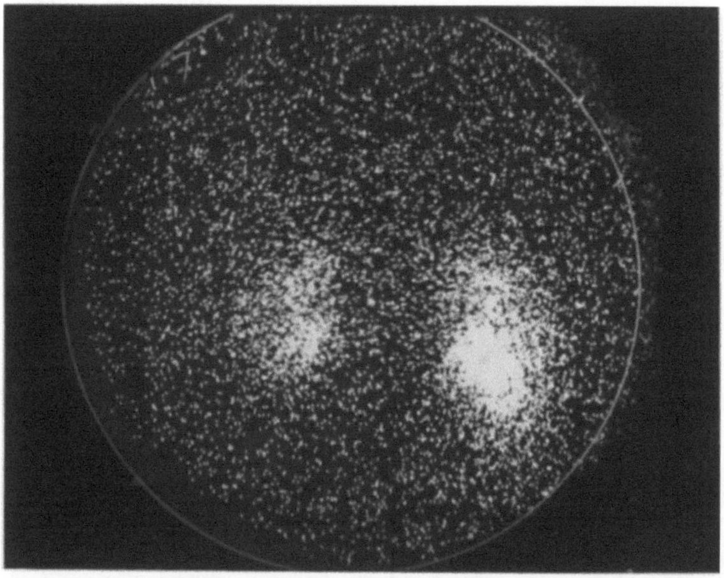

Fig. 25. The 0–3 min scintiphoto of 10-year-old female whose intravenous pyelogram is seen in Fig. 24. As is further demonstrated in Fig. 26, radionuclide uptake of right kidney is quite poor, yet quantitation is essential to assess exact function of this kidney

The patient had a right nephrectomy and repeat camera studies showed a 72% return, indicating complete and total compensatory hypertrophy on the left with no further urinary tract infections.

Without going into further detail concerning justification for surgical correction of reflux, it should be stated as the present feelings of this author that deterioration in kidney function and recurrent infection constitutes a clear-cut indication for intervention, usually surgically, but it should be pointed out that to our knowledge morphologic changes always are seen later and usually much later than functional changes. For this reason, we consider it exceedingly important to do frequent scintillation camera studies with adequate quantitation to evaluate the individual renal blood flow as well as the total renal blood flow.

The detection of vesicoureteral reflux traditionally has been done by urethral catheterization and injection of radiopaque media, and this probably is still the preferred choice, at least as an initial procedure for the demonstration of morphology. The use of radionuclides to demonstrate vesicoureteral reflux, however, has gained in popularity, primarily because of the reduced radiation dose associated with the use of radionuclides.

NAME S. F.

DATE 1.26. 1973

MATERIAL ^{131}I

SCINTILLATION CAMERA STUDY

TAPE # 16 PATIENT # 5782 SEX F AGE 9Y

BLOOD PRESSURE 100/68

PATIENT CONDITION HYDRATED

RECURRENT U.T.I.

TIME	R	%	L	%
0-1 COUNT	298	12	2234	88
CHANNEL	29	15	169	85
1-2	696	16	3593	84
	63	23	210	77
2-3	988	18	4377	82
	83	27	222	73
3-4	926	19	4029	81
	73	26	209	74
4-5	1028	24	3324	76
	79	32	171	68
10	1238	30	2882	70
	94	38	152	62
15	706	33	1468	67
	58	39	92	61
25	68	22	236	78
	6	27	22	73

MICROCURIES INJECTED 205

MICROCURIES EXCRETED IN 33 MINUTES

A) VOIDED 156 μci

B) RESIDUAL 0 μci

C) TOTAL 156 μci

URINE VOLUME 140 ML.

BLADDER COUNT IN 28 MINUTES 5997

BLADDER COUNT POST VOID 26

RESIDUAL URINE CALCULATED:

A) 0.4 %

B) 0 ML.

% OF RADIOHIPPURAN RETURNED IN 33 MIN.

A) VOIDED 76 %

B) RESIDUAL 0

C) TOTAL 76 %

****

STUDY DIAGNOSIS:

NORMAL ☐

ABNORMAL R ☐ L ☐ B ☐

SPECIFIC

M.D.

Fig. 26. Renal scintiphoto obtained with Radiohippuran showing full uptake on right. Print-outs of ^{131}I Hippuran scintillation camera study of child whose scintiphoto and intravenous pyelogram is seen in Fig. 25 and 24 respectively. It can be seen here that only 16% of total renal blood flow is present on right. Total renal blood flow is normal

The increasing use of radionuclide cystography is probably due to the ready availability of ^{99m}Tc pertechnetate and the low radiation dose despite using millicurie amounts. It has been estimated that at least 100 radionuclide studies can be performed before an equal amount of radiation is received as encountered with a single roentgenographic study.

BLAUFOX et al. in 1971 published their results with scintiphotography for the detection of vesicoureteral reflux in 47 children, utilizing ^{99m}Tc pertechnetate. Their method consists of instilling 500 μCi of ^{99m}Tc pertechnetate into the bladder, which is then distended gradually with saline. Utilizing an Anger camera, they record the distribution of radioactivity in the bladder and renal areas on Polaroid film during filling and overdistention of the bladder. They compared their technique with conventional radiographic cystourethrography and found good correlation between the two procedures. CONWAY et al. in 1974, reviewed the subject with a detailed description of their technique. They use 1 mCi of ^{99m}Tc pertechnetate of ^{99m}Tc sulfur colloid; the latter is supposed to decrease the chance of absorption of the radionuclide with subsequent secretion into the stomach. These authors find that the most significant levels of absorption occurred in those patients who were instrumented prior to the nuclear cystogram, even though such instrumentation was felt not to be traumatic.

SALVATIERRO et al. (1974) presented their studies utilizing ^{99m}Tc sulfur colloid particles for radionuclide cystography and recommend it for detection, study, and follow-up of vesicoureteral reflux. It is their feeling that the radionuclide cystography is more accurate and sensitive than x-ray cystography and has greater prognostic value. It is also their feeling that the ^{99m}Tc sulfur colloid particles better stimulate the movement of bacteria in the urinary tract, as was previously suggested by CORRIERE et al. (1967). A recent article by LIPSHULTZ and CORRIERE (1974) described the use of two radionuclides, i.e., ^{99m}Tc sulfur colloid and ^{131}I Hippuran. The colloid particles were suspended in the Radiohippuran solution and placed into the bladders of six patients. Three of these patients had a history of recurrent urinary tract infection, and they were found to eliminate the colloid particles at a much slower rate than the fluid. The authors suggest that a change in either the physical contour or secretory activity of the bladder urothelium is a possible cause of particle retention in these patients with chronic infections.

The low cost, the insignificant radiation exposure, and the ease of availability of ^{99m}Tc pertechnetate unquestionably makes the direct radionuclide cystography at least the method of choice for follow-up on children and adults with previously demonstrated reflux. The problem, however, does not get around the use of a urethral catheter. Indirect radionuclide cystography has been described but does not seem as yet to offer a practical answer, since it still incorporates that the patient must void upon command, which may be difficult if not impossible in infants and small children. Although such indirect radionuclide cystograms can be obtained in conjunction with a renal scintillation camera study utilizing

^{99m}Tc DTPA, problems are inherent with both radionuclides. The Radiohippuran, which is much more rapidly excreted, is given in much smaller dosages, thus giving very low count rates relative to those which can be obtained with ^{99m}Tc-labeled compounds. The latter, however, are handled primarily by filtration, and thus a substantial period of time has to be allowed to pass before the kidneys are empty. If ^{123}I-labeled Hippuran should become generally available, this may be the ideal radionuclide compound for indirect radionuclide cystography in the future.

L. Renal Tumors

Renal imaging for the purpose of detecting renal tumors has been popular ever since ^{203}Hg labeled chlormerodrin became available. Since chlormerodrin is fixed in the kidney, the use of the rectilinear scanner involving scanning time of approximately 45 min was of little consequence in regard to detecting cold spots in the kidneys. Due to the long physical half-life of ^{203}Hg and the subsequent relatively high radiation dose to the kidneys, ^{197}Hg chlormerodrin was subsequently used, and has today completely replaced ^{203}Hg.

With the availability of the gamma scintillation camera, ^{131}I labeled Hippuran and ^{99m}Tc are used extensively, either as additions to ^{197}Hg labeled chlormerodrin, or instead of the latter. The use of renal imaging for detection of tumors has its limitations, however, since it is unlikely that any tumors less than 2.5 cm in diameter can be detected by radionuclide imaging where the resolution can in no way compare with that obtained by a good radiologic study. It should, however, be remembered that many intravenous pyelograms done as screening procedures leave a lot to be desired, and although such procedures may be superior in demonstating a centrally located mass because of deformities or destruction of calyces, infundibula, or the renal pelvis, more peripheral cortical masses can better be demonstrated by renal imaging if proper radiopharmaceuticals are used.

A cold spot is, however, only indicative of a mass which is replacing normal functioning renal parenchyma and this may be representative of a cyst, a renal neoplasm which may be vascular or avascular, or an abscess. The renal imaging procedures can occasionally be exceedingly helpful in instances where a possible tumor appears present at intravenous urography. Apart from the previously mentioned cold spots, indicating decreased radioactivity, the occasional hot spots, imaging increased activity, can be useful in separating so-called renal pseudotumors from true tumors as seen, for instance, in prominent renal columns, which has been well described by BRAUNSTEIN et al. (1972) and POLLACK et al. (1974). According to these authors, a positive radionuclide finding should, in general, exclude the presence of a malignant neoplasm, and arteriography rarely is necessary to settle the question of true versus spurious masses raised by an equivocable urogram.

The attempts to use radionuclides and renal imaging to differentiate between renal neoplasm and cyst have been discussed and evaluated by numerous authors. GOTTA et al. (1973) and others, suggest that the presence or absence of intratumor blood supply can be used as a criteria for differential diagnosis of benign and malignant renal tumors. Two radiopharmaceuticals are used; chlormerodrin labeled with ^{203}Hg, which will show the tumor as a cold area, and this is then followed by ^{99m}Tc pertechnetate, which will show blood supply by initial blushing. Lack of blushing may be indicative of an avascular tumor. ROSENTHALL (1967) states that it is possible to distinguish neoplasm from cyst or ischemia by monitoring the kidneys with a gamma camera following a rapid intravenous injection of ^{99m}Tc pertechnetate. BLACK et al. (1968) also suggest the use of ^{203}Hg labeled chlormerodrin followed by ^{99m}Tc pertechnetate and stress the lack of morbidity and the accuracy of this diagnostic procedure. MORALES (1974), in discussing space occupying lesions of the kidney, emphasizes again the limitation of renal imaging in terms of the size of the lesion, and feels that the major contributions are in excluding the presence of tumors suspected from intravenous urograms and in studying the vascularity of a known lesion, provided the lesions are greater than 2.5 cm in diameter. He recommends the use of ^{99m}Tc iron ascorbate because of the higher count rate, the smaller radiation dose, and less photon attenuation than with ^{197}Hg chlormerodrin. He does, however, suggest that the initial static view should be done with ^{197}Hg chlormerodrin and emphasizes that the technique does not allow the physician to distinguish between a cyst, an abscess, and an avascular solid tumor.

The use of radionuclides and renal imaging in the diagnosis of space-occupying lesions in the kidney seems advantageous to radiographic procedures only if the patient has a previous history of reaction to contrast media, or as a possible supplementary evaluation of suspected lesions on intravenous urography. Attempting to distinguish between a cyst on the one hand and a neoplasm on the other hand is probably only advantageous in the poor risk patient, provided that such diagnostic procedures can be combined with ultrasonic scanning for further evaluation of the nature of the space-occupying lesion. It also should be pointed out that it is not uncommon to have a relatively clear-cut cold spot on a Radiohippuran scintiphoto or a ^{99m}Tc DTPA scintiphoto, where an intravenous urogram may not reveal any lesion. Consequently, we feel that it is entirely possible to rule out the presence of space-occupying lesions greater than approximately 2.5 cm when the Radiohippuran scintillation camera studies are done as routine screening procedures. If, however, a patient presents with hematuria, any possible radionuclide imaging procedure should probably be done only as an additional diagnostic approach, with intravenous urography and/or nephrotomography as well as renal angiography being essential for providing morphologic details. The additional use of ultrasonic scanning as well as possible cyst puncture with injection of radiopaque media are other commonly used diagnostic procedures.

It has been previously stated that the utilization of the gamma scintillation camera with ability to quantitate individual renal blood flow as well as blood flow within the kidney perhaps constitutes a more important aspect of the utilization of radionuclides in urology than does imaging, and such also holds true when dealing with renal tumors. To the surgeon, it is of paramount importance to know the exact state of the contralateral normal kidney as well as the total kidney function, and as illustrated in Fig. 27, 28, and 29, the removal of a kidney with a normal contralateral mate which had only approximately 15% of the total function, revealed surprisingly a large hypernephroma which was not apparent from either the intravenous pyelogram or from the angiogram. The fact, however, that the kidney function was so poor without any obvious sign of obstruction made it a relatively simple surgical decision, even though the preoperative diagnosis was by no means certain.

The use of radionuclides in renal imaging for diagnosis of neoplasm has so far been primarily one of cold spots indicating lack of parenchymal uptake except for blood flow studies utilizing ^{99m}Tc pertechnetate. However, Kaplan et al. (1974) have described increased activity in a renal tubular adenoma. Various radiopharmaceuticals have been used and are still being used in an attempt to obtain specific localization of tumor resulting from a higher concentration and accumulation in tumor tissue and such agents have included Bleomycin as described by Grove et al. (1974), Gallium as reported by Langhammer et al. (1972), and ^{167}Tm, ^{169}Yb, and ^{175}Yb in the citrate form as suggested by Hisada et al. (1974), and recently as described by Hoffer et al. (personal communica-

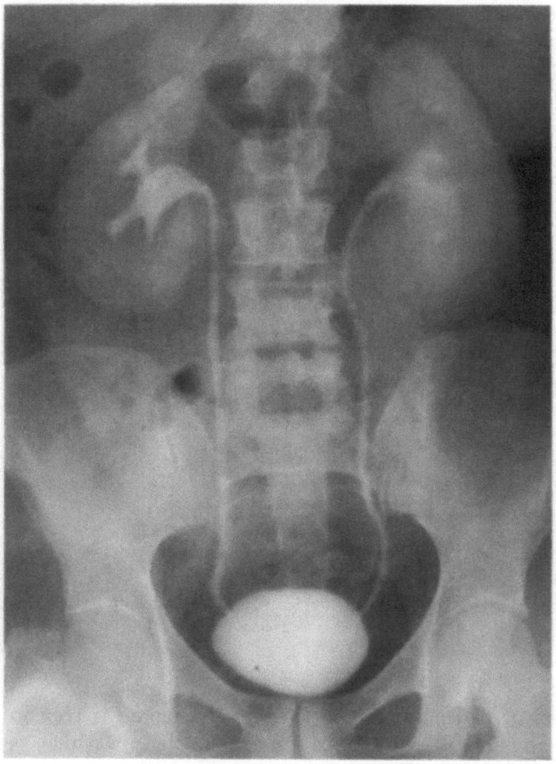

Fig. 27. Intravenous pyelogram showing poor contrast in collecting system on left but no obvious tumor masses

tion), use of radioiodinated antibodies specific for the carcinoembryonic antigen produced by the tumor has shown some promising results.

The utilization of specific organ imaging can be helpful in delineating tumors of the upper pole of the kidney or suprarenal masses. We often do combined imaging of liver and spleen with ^{99m}Tc sulfur colloid and ^{131}I Hippuran as seen in Fig. 30, and in instances of subdiaphragmatic masses, transmission images with ^{57}Co or lung images with ^{99m}Tc iron hydroxide aggregates will allow a spacial evaluation showing displacement of the diaphragm, liver, or spleen.

As seen on Fig. 30, the normal close proximity of the spleen and the left kidney is occupied by a cold area, which proved to be an adrenal cyst. The list of useful approaches utilizing radionuclide imaging in detecting or evaluating renal masses is seemingly endless, and undoubtedly new methods will develop, and resolution will improve. Presently, however, renal imaging for diagnosis of renal tumors must be considered supplementary to radiological studies.

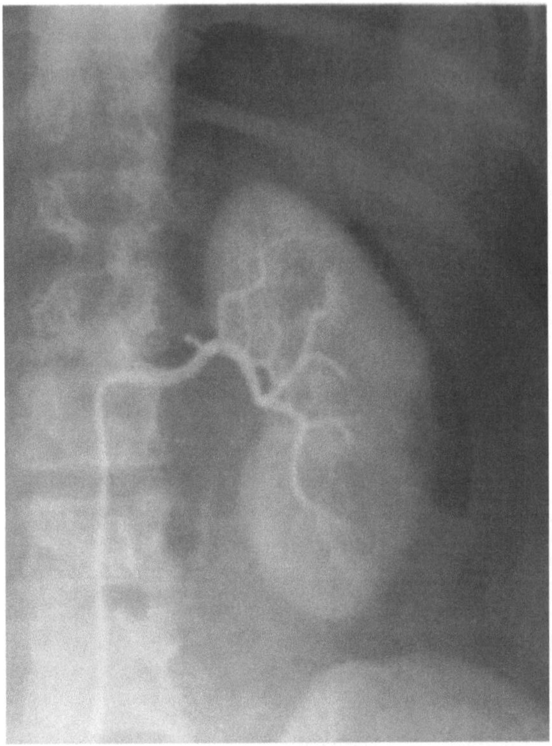

Fig. 28. Angiogram of patient whose intravenous pyelogram is seen in Fig. 27, showing no tumor stain in any area. Renal scintillation camera study was then performed (Fig. 29)

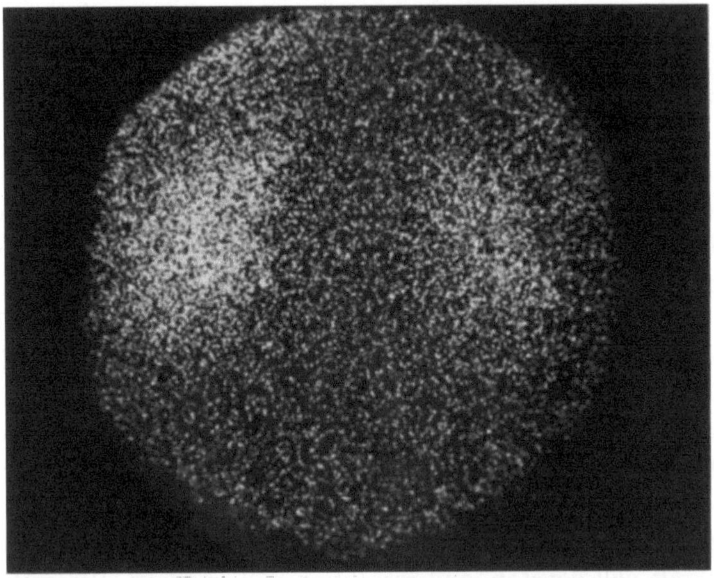

Fig. 29. Scintiphoto presented here shows poor uptake on left with calculated blood flow that amounted to no more than 15% of total. Patient was found to have large hypernephroma of kidney occupying entire lower two-thirds

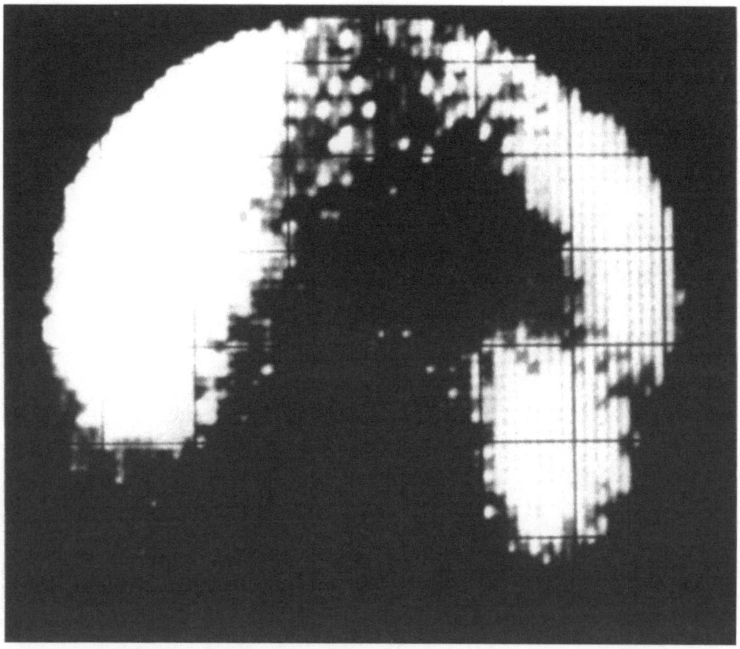

Fig. 30. Scintillation camera imaging of liver, spleen, and both kidneys shows obvious cold area between upper pole of left kidney and spleen which at surgery was proven to be occupied by large adrenal cyst

M. Injuries

One area in which scintiphotography appears to have an enormous potential involves its use in the acutely injured patient. Unfortunately Gamma cameras have not yet made their entry in large numbers in the emergency room setting, but it is difficult to see why it should not be one of the most important tools for evaluating trauma to internal organs. As stated by BERG (1974), imaging studies utilizing the dynamic and static capabilities of the scintillation camera are uniquely suited to the need for rapid, noninvasive, and reliable examination of the acutely traumatized patient. Of 973 acutely traumatized patients whom he examined, they found splenic trauma in 118, lacerated livers in 57, and renal trauma in 52 patients. A large number of these patients had renal trauma associated with splenic injury. There are today available portable cameras, as shown in Fig. 31, which allow studies to be done without moving the patient to the camera, but rather by moving the camera to the patient.

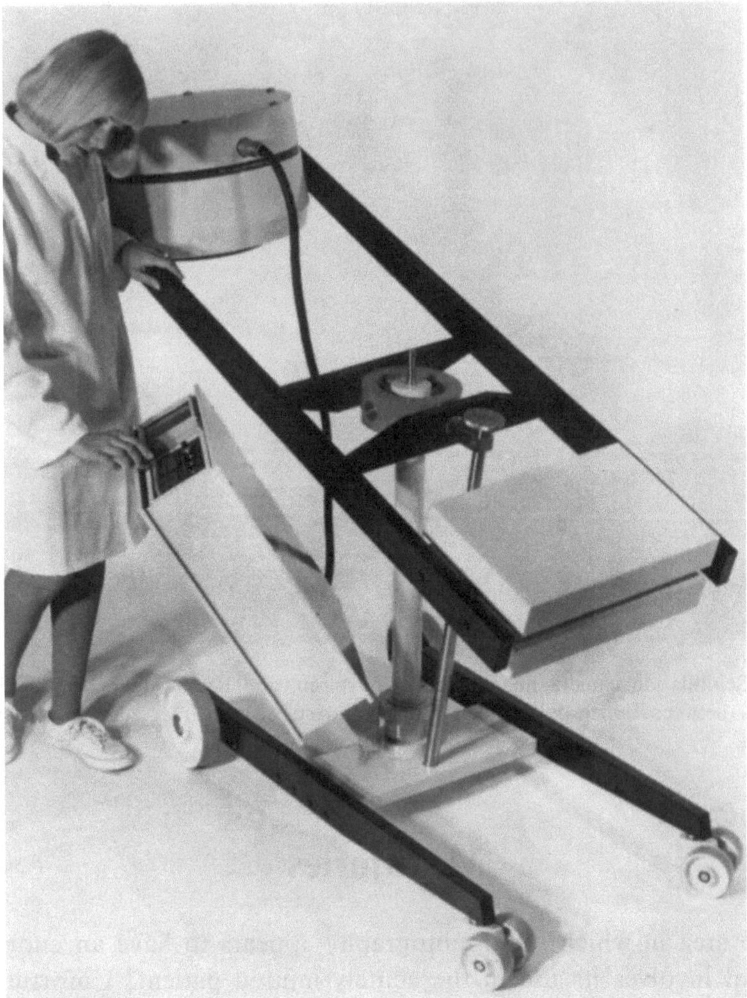

Fig. 31. New light-weight portable gamma scintillation camera designed exclusively for studies utilizing ^{99m}Tc or radionuclides with KEV in same range

The "immediate management/care protocol" described by BERG (1974) and as performed at the St. Francis Hospital, University of Illinois, deserves quotation:

Since rapid diagnosis is essential to the management and care of the acutely traumatized patient, a protocol has been established to fulfill this condition. Upon arrival of the patient in the emergency room, he is placed upon a Surgilift carrier or other special type conveyance that will minimize further movement. The nuclear medicine division is immediately notified to be ready when the patient's condition becomes stable. Either an intravenous infusion is started or a cut-down is performed. In the emergency room, radiography of the chest, thoracic cage, and abdomen is obtained. These are evaluated by the radiologist in charge of nuclear medicine. With the clinical laboratory and radiographic information then available, the appropriate nuclear medicine procedures, if required, can be selected. If multiple studies are indicated, the proper sequence is chosen on the basis of the condition of the patient and primary organ system involved. If primary liver or spleen injury is suspected, the hepatosplenic imaging study will be performed first. If splenic injury is thereby demonstrated, the renovascular flow and imaging examination is usually added. The reason for this is the high incidence of renal injury in association with splenic trauma in our experience. If renal injury seems not only most likely but of paramount clinical importance, the renovascular flow and imaging study is the initial procedure of choice. If renal injury is found or is suspected on the dynamic and initial static imaging stages of the examination, an infusion urogram is instituted during the period between the three serial immediate static and delayed (1 h) static images.

For evaluation of renal trauma it appears presently that images obtained by injection of ^{99m}Tc DTPA in bolus with flow studies as well as imaging is exceedingly useful to evaluate possible traumatic renal artery thrombosis as well as laceration of the renal parenchyma. Traumatic renal artery thrombosis as discussed by SKINNER (1973) requires prompt recognition of the lesion and immediate surgical intervention. In such patients, nearly 50% had no clinical evidence of major intra-abdominal or retroperitoneal injury and scintillation camera studies as described by HARTENBOWER et al. (1970) should allow prompt recognition of arterial occlusion, thus permitting early revascularization attempts. The previously mentioned combination with imaging of the spleen has been discussed by NEBESAR et al. (1974), who recommended it as a primary method of evaluation for possible splenic trauma, with angiography reserved for unusual or equivocable cases, an opinion shared by LUCEY and SMITH (1973), who examined 16 patients with abdominal trauma and screened them for possible spleen injury. It was their feeling that angiography probably is not needed if the spleen scintigram is negative. KOENIGSBERG et al. (1974) feel that roentgenographic and radionuclide investigation are indicated in all patients with gross or microscopic hematuria after trauma. They recommend that the initial studies should include high dose infusion urography and static renal scintigraphy. If both examinations are within normal limits, no further work-up may be necessary. It is their recommendation that if no contrast media appears in the kidney during urography, a radiopertechnetate flow study should be done. If there is no renal activity during this study, this would be suggestive of a major arterial occlusion and thus prompt renal angiography should be performed.

Major and minor renal injury can, according to these authors, be distinguished by follow-up radionuclide imaging studies since infarcts

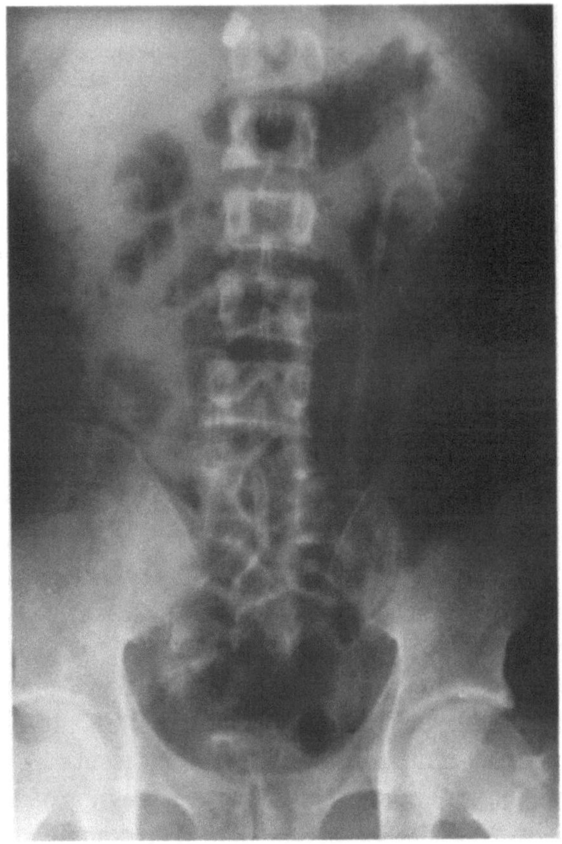

Fig. 32. Intravenous pyelogram from 21-year-old male who sustained gunshot wound to right flank, showing faint nephrogram on right with evidence of extravasation

will remain with persistent defects while contusions will demonstrate a return to a normal pattern over the following weeks. Their experience indicates that when the radionuclide study has been normal, no significant injuries have been observed on angiographic examination. It is their recommendation that the safety and ease of performance make the radionuclide technique of great value initially as well as for serial follow-up studies.

The following case is that of a 21-year-old male who sustained a gunshot wound to the right flank and presented with gross hematuria. As seen in Fig. 32, there is a faint nephrogram on the right, with evidence of extravasation. The renal scintillation camera study (Fig. 33) shows evidence of decreased function, especially in an area corresponding to the laceration found at surgery across the posterior aspect of the right kidney.

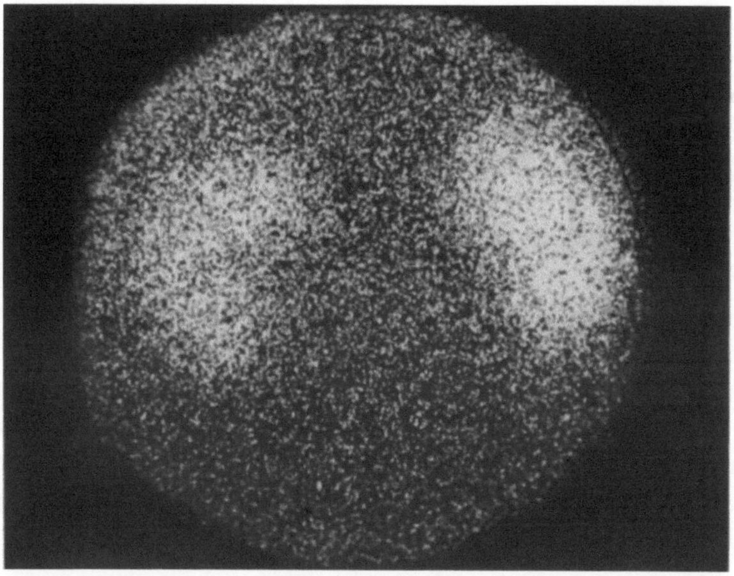

Fig. 33. Renal scintiphoto with ^{131}I Hippuran shows decreased uptake of right lower pole and specifically in area below middle of right kidney corresponding to area damaged by path of bullet

FREEMAN (1973) feels that renal scintiphotography can be used as a screening technique in cases of injury and infarction of the kidney where the urogram notoriously is nonspecific for such situations. He suggests the use of ^{197}Hg chlormerodrin in traumatic lesions, where the image can depict focal areas of injury which can be followed with serial studies. It is his experience that such findings on the radiochlormerodrin study correlate well with angiography. The use of radiopertechnetate and ^{131}I-labeled Hippuran is recommended if the patient is suspected of having embolic renovascular disease or where questions exist on any of the other scintillation camera studies.

Unfortunately, a systematic use of radionuclides and organ imaging in cases of trauma is not yet the order of the day, but to quote BERG.

> The imaging techniques should be available at the community hospital level by those regional hospitals equipped and staffed for the emergency care of the traumatized patient.

With adequate renal blood flow and the use of ^{131}I Hippuran, urinary extravasation by rupture of the renal pelvis, ureters, or bladder can readily be assessed on follow-up scintiphotos, so that further radiologic studies can be undertaken for better morphologic details. Certainly a normal renal imaging with two equally well functioning kidneys and no indication of urinary extravasation makes it reasonably safe to assume that no injury to the urinary tract has occurred, and the ease and safety of the examination should make it *sine qua non*.

N. Miscellaneous Subjects

I. Testes

Testicular imaging with ^{99m}Tc pertechnetate has been suggested by several authors as a useful technique to distinguish between torsion of the testicle and epididymitis. If the scintiphoto shows lack of perfusion on the affected side, as indicated by a cold area, this is strongly suggestive of torsion of the testicle.

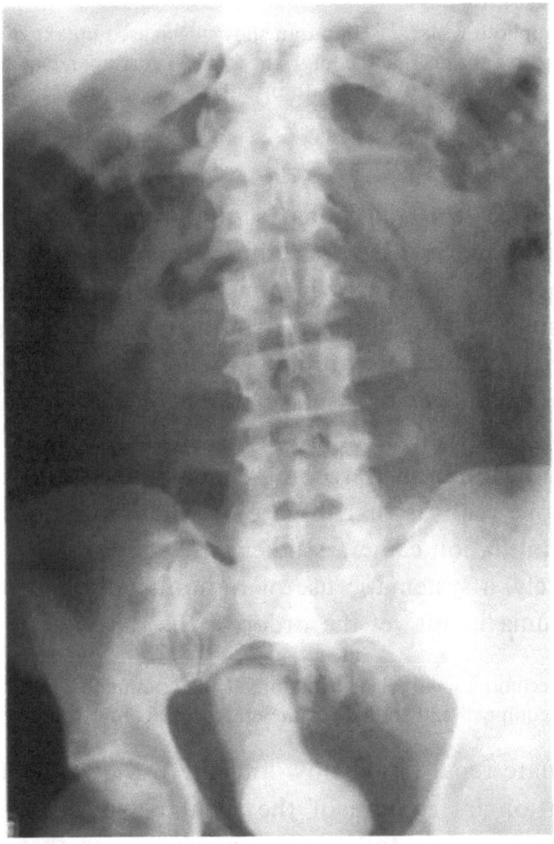

Fig. 34. Intravenous pyelogram 20 min after injection, which in previous films had demonstrated no function of left and normal kidney on right, shows bladder filling with obvious displacement of bladder to right

II. Prostate

ANDERSSON et al. (1967) has suggested the use of ^{133}Xe for measurement of prostatic blood flow, and we recently attempted with ^{99m}Tc pertechnetate to evaluate a large prostate with a suspected prostatic abscess. In the latter case, a large cold area confirmed the suspicion of prostatic abscess, which was consequently proven by incision and drainage.

As illustrated by the following case, gallium can at times be useful to show metastatic tumor of prostatic origin. A 62-year-old male presented with a several months' history of swelling of his left lower extremity along with vague lower abdominal pain. An intravenous pyelogram, as illustrated in Fig. 34, showed no function on the left and a displacement of the bladder to the right. Rectal examination revealed an enlarged prostate of reasonably normal consistency. Serum acid phosphatase was on several occasions elevated and a left retrograde pyelogram

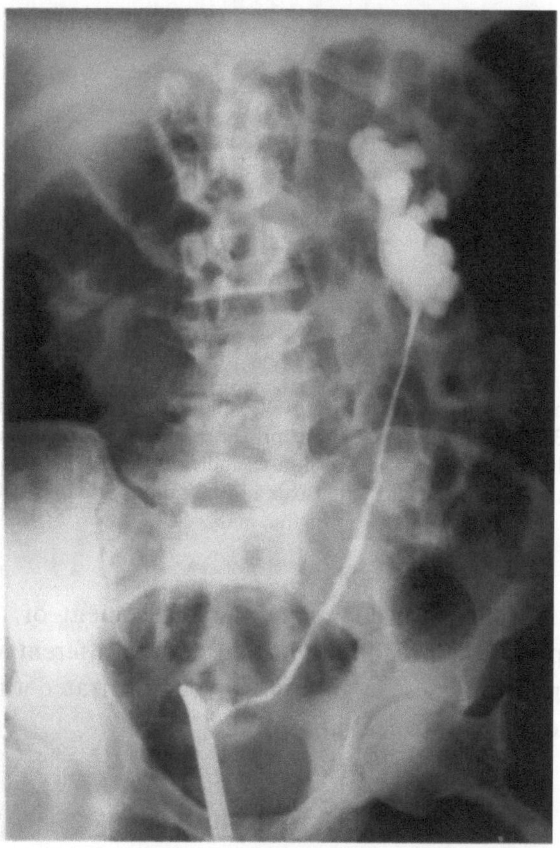

Fig. 35. Retrograde pyelogram on patient whose intravenous pyelogram appears in Fig. 34, with displacement of bladder to right, indicating displacement of ureter to left with corresponding displacement of pelvis and ureteropelvic junction

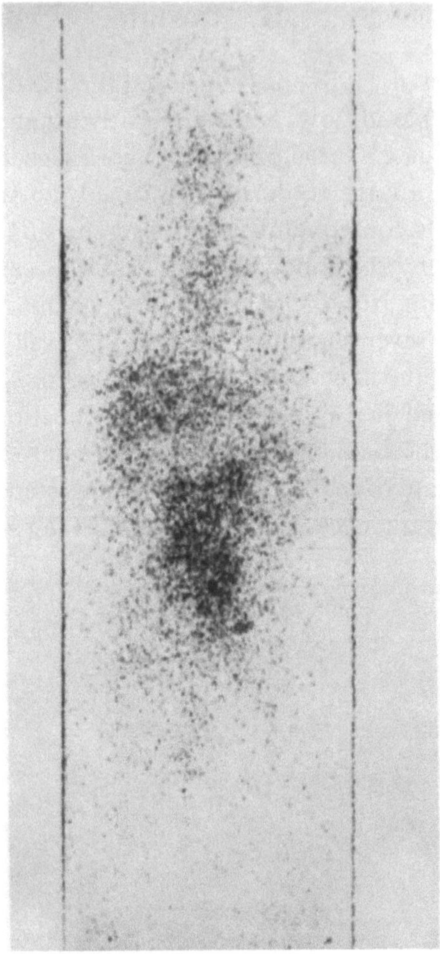

Fig. 36. Gallium scan from patient whose IVP and retrograde pyelogram were depicted in Fig. 34 and 35 respectively, and whose prostatic biopsy showed poorly differentiated carcinoma. Gallium scan shows uptake in area indicative of tumor mass which displaced bladder to right and left ureter to left. Liver can be faintly visualized above and to right of this mass

as shown in Fig. 35 showed a lateral displacement of the left ureter. A needle biopsy of the prostate indicated poorly differentiated carcinoma and a gallium scan, as seen in Fig. 36, demonstrated the large tumor present in the retroperitoneal area.

III. Adrenals

Adrenal tumors have been evaluated with radionuclides. BLAIR et al. (1971) suggested the use of radio-labeled cholesterol, which in some adrenal tumors presented as a hot spot, and HURWITZ et al. (1973), utilizing ^{131}I-19-iodocholesterol, published its use in two patients, where it localized in functional adrenocortical tumors. STURMAN et al. (1974) has advocated the use of Radiocholesterol for the localization of pheochromocytomas; however, the radionuclide does not seem to localize in the pheochromocytoma itself, yet the affected adrenal was correctly identified preoperatively in 6 patients by either absence of or decreased activity. FITZER (1974) published a case report of a 9-month-old girl who presented with a hard lobulated mass extending from the right costal margin to the right lower quadrant. As part of her work-up a ^{99m}Tc polyphosphate bone scan was performed, and an intense concentration of the radiopharmaceutical was found in the right upper quadrant mass. The mass was found to be an adrenal neuroblastoma and whether the nonosseous uptake was secondary to abundant calcification throughout the tumor, or whether there was a specific affinity for the neuroblastoma, is unresolved.

IV. Bone

The terminology "bone scan" is correct even though today most commonly a gamma scintillation camera is used; however, it is moved in a set pattern, and thus the resulting imaging of the skeletal system is indeed a scan. The urologist has more than a fleeting interest in the abnormalities encountered in bone scans, as it results from disseminated prostatic carcinoma, hypernephroma, hyperparathyroidism, as well as any possible other metastatic lesions from the genitourinary system to the skeletal system. The most popular radionuclide for bone scanning presently appears to be ^{99m}Tc labeled to polyphosphate. This seems to have replaced ^{18}F in skeletal radionuclide scanning (BARRETT and SMITH, 1974; and WEBER et al., 1974).

Bone lesions can be "cold" or "hot." GOERGEN et al. (1974) reports on cold bone lesions, and described findings in seven patients with a variety of disease processes, including metastatic disease, posttraumatic aseptic necrosis, and sickle cell crisis, studied with ^{99m} Tc polyphosphate and ^{18}F scans. They further studied two cases with ^{111}In chloride bone marrow scans. They identified foci of decreased radionuclide activity corresponding to sites of metastatic tumors and bone infarcts. The use of bone scan in primary hyperthyroidism has been described by SY (1974), who found that the bone scan abnormalities were not unlike the distribution of abnormally decreased activity of dialysis patients with a secondary type. He recommends the use of ^{99m}Tc labeled polyphosphate in patients with hypercalcemia or suspected hyperthyroidism.

In Paget's disease, MILLER et al. (1974) have described the procedure using ^{99m}Tc polyphosphate in 25 patients and found it useful to evaluate the extent of the lesion, which may be difficult to judge by roentgenographic means. SHEARER et al. (1974) reported on their experience with x-rays, ^{87m}Sr scintigraphy, and ^{99m}Tc polyphosphate scintigraphy in the identification of bone metastases in 201 patients with prostatic cancer. They had about 40% of the patients demonstrating metastases in the bone the first time they were seen. The results of their study showed that using x-ray and ^{87m}Sr, x-rays failed to detect metastasis in 10% of the cases where they were identified by the ^{87m}Sr, but the radionuclide survey similarly failed to detect radiologic evidence of deposits in 7% of the cases.

In similar studies comparing ^{99m}Tc polyphosphate scans with x-ray surveys, the x-ray surveys missed radionuclide-detected metastasis in 12% of cases reported, but only in 1 case out of 67 did the radionuclide study miss radiologically evident deposits. In 32 patients investigated by the radionuclide techniques with ^{99m}Tc polyphosphate, none failed to detect any metastasis and identified deposit in 1 patient in whom it was missed by ^{87m}Sr scintigraphy. About 15% of x-ray and ^{87m}Sr surveys have equivocable results, but only 3% of the ^{99m}Tc polyphosphate surveys were equivocal. It was their feeling that the ^{99m}Tc polyphosphate bone scanning utilizing a gamma camera was the most reliable of the techniques used for identification of bone metastases in patients with carcinoma of the prostate.

In a paper by KAPLAN et al. (1974), also using ^{99m}Tc polyphosphate in patients with histologically proven neoplastic involvement of the skeleton, the scan performed 5 h after intravenous administration showed only a subtle increase in activity while at 10 h the concentration of activity relative to background was greatly enhanced. A number of other publications attest to the value of the use of ^{99m}Tc polyphosphate for bone imaging and since this radiopharmaceutical generally visualized the kidneys with reasonably good definition, a bonus appears as reported by MANDEL et al. (1974) and JACKMAN et al. (1974), where unsuspected renal tumors or abnormalities became apparent by viewing the renal imaging as a part of the total body scan. In this connection it should also be realized that for proper evaluation of the bony pelvis, the bladder should be empty since a high concentration will occur in the urine, thus obscuring abnormalities in the bony structures of the pelvis.

V. Lungs

The important aspect of lung imaging to the urologist is to attempt to differentiate between pulmonary emboli and other pathologic states which may confuse the diagnosis. The utilization of radionuclides in this area is still very much in its infancy, although some information can be obtained which adds to the information obtained by a chest radiograph and possibly angiography. As pointed out by SECKER-WALKER and SIEGEL (1973), the two studies are complementary, one showing the anatomical location of the thrombi and the other, the functional disturbances caused by them.

Camera imaging of the lungs according to these investigators should preferably be performed with ^{99m}Tc-labeled particles and it is their feeling that albumin macroaggregates or microspheres are a better choice than ferric hydroxide particles. Since the results of such studies primarily deal with blood flow, they suggest that aerosol scans be added to the diagnostic armamentarium. A number of radiopharmaceuticals have been used for this purpose and without going into detail in regard to the advantages or disadvantages, it should be merely pointed out that this procedure may help in distinguishing between pulmonary embolism and atelectasis in addition to chest radiography and possibly angiography. It appears at the present time that the lung imaging is helpful but not diagnostic in the acute situation, yet for follow-up studies it may provide an extremely useful therapeutic guide.

VI. Thrombophlebitis

As a continuation of the problems facing the surgeon where pulmonary emboli versus atelectasis or other pulmonary complications are vital, the diagnosis of thrombophlebitis, especially in the upper thigh and pelvis, is of utmost importance. WEBBER et al. (1974) have used macroaggregated albumin entrapment in areas of fibrin deposits to detect intravenous thrombosis. They have compared the uptake with venography and autologous ^{125}I labeled fibrinogen uptake in approximately 30 cases. It is their conclusion that the macroaggregated albumin labeled with ^{99m}Tc appears very accurate in locating thromboses in the upper thigh and pelvis, where fibrinogen uptake is less helpful. They expressed the feeling that the correlation suggests that the macroaggregated albumin labeled with ^{99m}Tc gives very few false-negative results and that the procedure is easily performed in conjunction with a perfusion lung scan.

CHARKES et al. (1974) reported on the use of ^{131}I fibrinogen for the detection of deep vein thrombosis using the gamma scintillation camera. In 29 postoperative patients, 8 of whom had a fractured hip, ^{131}I fibrinogen was injected and whole body scintiscans were made at frequent intervals for a week. They performed venograph in 20 of the patients and the concurrence between the two studies was 93%. It is their feeling that scintiscanning with ^{131}I fibronogen had certain advantages over the ^{125}I fibrinogen method, including the possibility of detecting iliac vein thrombi.

References

Adam, W.E., Kadatz, R., Bitter, F., Sigmund, E., Wack, H.O.: Investigations on kidney perfusion tests with radioactive substances. In: Radionuclides in Nephrology (Blaufox, M.D. and Funck-Bretano, J.-L., eds.), pp. 341–349. New York: Grune & Stratton 1972.

Anderson, C.F., Sawyer, T.K., Cutler, R.E.: Iothalamate Sodium 1–125 vs. Cyanocobalamin Co-57 as a measure of glomerular filtration rate in man. J. Amer. med. Ass. **204**, 653–656 (1968).

Anderson, T., McDowell, T., Jr., Mintzer, R.A., Hoffer, P.B., Lusted, L.B., Smith, V.C., Pokorny, J.: Nuclear image transmission by picturephone evaluation by ROC curve method. Invest. Radiol. **8**, 244–250 (1973).

Andersson, L., Dahn, I., Nelson, C.-E., Norgren, A.: Method for measuring prostatic blood flow with $Xenon^{133}$ in the dog. Invest. Urol. **5**, 140–148 (1967).

Anger, H.O.: Scintillation camera with multichannel collimators. J. nucl. Med. **5**, 515–531 (1964).

Arimizu, N., Morris, A.C., Jr.: Quantitative measurement of radioactivity in internal organs by area scanning. J. nucl. Med. **10**, 265–269 (1969).

Arruda, J.A.L., Boonjarern, Sampanta, Westenfelder, Ch., Kurtzman, N.A.: Measurement of renal blood flow with radioactive microspheres. Proc. Soc. exp. Biol. (N.Y.) **146**, 263–264 (1974).

Ashburn, W.L., Harbert, J.C., Whitehouse, W.C., Mason, D.T.: A video system for recording dynamic radioisotope studies with the Anger scintillation camera. J. nucl. Med. **9**, 554–561 (1968).

Atkins, H.L., Freeman, L.M.: The investigation of renal disease using radionuclides. Postgrad. med. J. **49**, 503–516 (1973).

Awad, W., Bennett, L.R., Martin, D.C.: Detection of renal homograft rejection reaction with a single dose of radiohippuran. J. Urol. (Baltimore) **100**, 233–237 (1968).

Baitz, T., Hallenbeck, G.A., Shorter, R.G., Scott, G.W., Owen, Ch.A., Jr., Hunt, J.C.: Preservation of kidneys for transplantation. Arch. Surg. **91**, 276–287 (1965).

Bankir, L., Grunfeld, J.P.: Intrarenal distribution of blood flow measured in unanesthetized rabbits with the Krypton 85 method. In: Radionuclides in Nephrology (Blaufox, M.D. and Funck-Bretano, J.-L., eds.), pp. 21–22. New York: Grune & Stratton 1972.

Barger, A.C.: Measurement of the distribution of intrarenal blood flow in the chronic, unanesthetized dog. In: Radionuclides in Nephrology (Blaufox, M.D. and Funck-Bretano, J.-L., eds.), pp. 3–7. New York: Grune & Stratton 1972.

Barrett, J.J., Smith, P.H.S.: Bone Imaging with $^{99}Tc^{m}$ Polyphosphate: A Comparison with ^{18}F and Skeletal Radiography. Brit. J. Radiol. **47**, 387–392 (1974).

Beierwaltes, W., Sturman, M.F., Ryo, U., Ice, R.D.: Imaging functional nodules of the adrenal glands with ^{131}I-19-iodocholesterol. J. nucl. Med. **15**, 246–251 (1974).

Beihn, R.M., Damron, J.R., Hafner, T.: Subtraction technique for the detection of subphrenic abscesses using ^{67}Ga and ^{99m}Tc. J. nucl. Med. **15**, 371–373 (1974).

Berg, B.C., Jr.: Radionuclide studies after urinary-tract injury. Semin. nucl. Med. **4**, 371–393 (1974).

Bernstein, L.H., Schlegel, J.U., O'Dell, R.M.: Differential renograms for evaluation of renal tubular function. Surg. Forum **18**, 533–535 (1967).

Bianchi, C.: Measurement of the glomerular filtration rate. In: Progress in Nuclear Medicine, Chapter 3, Volume 2 (Blaufox, M.D., ed.), pp. 21–53. Baltimore: University Park Press 1972.

Bianchi, C., Blaufox, M.D.: ^{131}I-hypaque and ^{140}La-DTPA for the measurement of glomerular filtration rate in dog. J. nucl. Biol. Med. **12**, 117–120 (1968).

Bianchi, C., Coli, A., Meozzi, A., Protto, C., Palla, R.: A. New methods of measuring glomerular filtration: The glomerular filtration rate in clinical practice. The reliability of the Hypaque-I^{131} and external counting method. Excerpta med., Int. Congr. Ser. No 178, 161–164 (1967).

Bianchi, C., Coli, A., Palla, R., LoMoro, A.: The reliability of ^{140}La-DTPA for the determination of glomerular filtration rate in man. J. nucl. Biol. Med. **17** (4), 158–161 (1973).

Bianchi, C., Coli, A., Palla, R., Rindi, P.: Divided renal plasma flow measurement: the improvement of a new technique. Excerpta med., Int. Congress Ser. No 178, 273–277 (1967).

Black, M.B., King, Ch.D., Smith, D.R.: Double Isotope scintiphotography for differentiating between renal cysts and renal tumors. J. Urol. (Baltimore) **98**, 728–734 (1968).

Blair, R.J., Beierwaltes, W.H., Lieberman, L.M., Boyd, Ch.M., Counsell, R.E., Weinhold, P.A., Varma, V.M.: Radiolabeled cholesterol as an adrenal scanning agent. J. nucl. Med. **12**, 176–182 (1971).

Blau, M.: An answer to the AEC on ^{197}Hg Chlormerodrin. J. nucl. Med. **9**, 206–207 (1968).

Blaufox, M.D.: Measurement of renal function with radioactive materials. In: Progress in Nuclear Medicine, Chapter 2, Volume 2 (Blaufox, M.D., ed.), pp. 9–20. Baltimore: University Park Press 1972.

Blaufox, M.D.: Methods for measurement of the renal blood flow. In: Progress in Nuclear Medicine, Chapter 5, Volume 2 (Blaufox, M.D., ed.), pp. 21–84. Baltimore: University Park Press 1972.

Blaufox, M.D.: The normal renogram: A. Compartment analysis of the radiorenogram and kinetics of ^{131}Hippuran. In: Progress in Nuclear Medicine, Chapter 7, Volume 2 (Blaufox, M.D., ed.), pp. 107–124. Baltimore: University Park Press 1972.

Blaufox, M.D.: The normal renogram: C. Determination of residual urine. In: Progress in Nuclear Medicine, Chapter 7, Volume 2 (Blaufox, M.D., ed.), pp. 138–142. Baltimore: University Park Press 1972.

Blaufox, M.D.: Scintigraphy in diseases of the urinary tract: C. Vesicoureteral reflux. In: Progress in Nuclear Medicine, Chapter 13, Volume 2 (Blaufox, M.D., ed.), pp. 289–295. Baltimore: University Park Press 1972.

Blaufox, M.D., Cohen, A.: Single-injection clearances of iothalamate-^{131}I in rats. Amer. J. Physiol. **218**(2), 542–544 (1970).

Blaufox, M.D., Conroy, N.F.: Measurement of renal mass transit time of Hippuran^{131} with external counting. J. nucl. Bio. Med. **12**, 107 (1968).

Blaufox, M.D., Fromowitz, A., Meng, C.-H., Lee, H.B., Elkin, M.: Renal blood flow and renin activity in renal venous blood in essential hypertension. Circulat. Res. **27**, 913–920 (1970).

Blaufox, M.D., Grushkin, A., Sandler, P., Goldman, H., Ogwo, J.E., Edelmann, Ch.M.: Radionuclide scintigraphy for detection of vesicoureteral reflux in children. J. Pediat. **79**, 239–246 (1971).

Blaufox, M.D., Guttman, R.D., Merill, J.P.: Measurement of renal function in the rat with single injection clearances. Amer. J. Physiol. **212**, 243–246 (1968).

Blaufox, M.D., Merrill, J.P.: Simplified hippuran clearance: 1. Measurement of renal function in man with simplified hippuran clearances. Nephron **3**, 274–281 (1966).

Blaufox, M.D., Potchen, E., Merill, J.P.: Measurement of effective renal plasma flow in man by external counting methods. J. nucl. Med. **8**, 77–85 (1967).

Block, J.B., Rieselbach, R.E., Bentzel, C.J., Rall, D.P.: Comparison of measurements of renal function by an external monitoring technique and renal clearance. Proc. Soc. exp. Biol. (N.Y.) **117**, 297 (1964).

Botti, R.E., Razzak, M.A., McIntyre, W.J., Pritchard, W.H.: The relationship of renal blood flow to cardiac output in normal individuals as determined by concomitant radioisotopic measurements. Cardiovasc. Res. **2**, 243–246 (1968).

Boyd, R.E., Robson, J., Hunt, F.C., Sorby, P.J., Murray, I.P.C., McKay, W.J.: $^{99}Tc^{m}$ gluconate complexes for renal scintigraphy. Brit. J. Radiol. **46**, 604–612 (1973).

Braunstein, P., Hernberg, J.G., Bosniak, M.A., Barasch, E.: Scintiscan evaluation of prominent renal columns. Radiology **104**, 103–106 (1972).

Brien, T.G., Fay, J.A.: ^{51}Cr-EDTA biological half-life as an index of renal function. J. nucl. Med. **13**, 339–340 (1972).

Brown, D.W.: Digital computer analysis and display of the radioisotope scan. J. nucl. Med. **5**, 802–806 (1964).

Brown, N.J.G., Britton, K.E.: The theory of renography and analysis of results. In: Radionuclides in Nephrology (Blaufox, M.D. and Funck-Bretano, J.-L., eds.), pp. 315–324. New York: Grune & Stratton 1972.

Bueschen, A.J., Evans, B.B., Schlegel, J.U.: Renal scintillation camera studies in children. J. Urol. (Baltimore) **111**, 821–824 (1974).

Burke, G., Halko, A.: Dynamic clinical studies with radioisotopes and the scintillation camera: Sodium iodohippurate I^{131} renography employing electronic crystal splitting. Amer. J. Roentgenol. **6**, 792–800 (1967).

Burke, G., Halko, A.: Scintillation camera renography in the study of prolonged transit time. Radiology **88**, 704–712 (1967).

Byrom, H., Dean, P.M., Sear, R., Turnbull, A.L., Tresidder, G.C., Blandy, J.P.: Technical improvements in renal scanning. Proc. roy. Soc. Med. **63**, 331–336 (1970).

Cangiano, J.L., Genuth, S.M., Renerts, L., Berman, L.N.: Simplified measurement of glomerular filtration rate. Invest. Urol. **9**, 34–38 (1971).

Cantraine, F.R.L., Bergmann, P., Greens, M., Lenaers, A., Jank, K., Cleempoel, H.: A quantitative description of the radiorenogram based on the arteriovenous and arterio-urinary weighting functions. In: Radionuclides in Nephrology (Blaufox, M.D. and Funck-Bretano, J.-L., eds.), pp. 333–340. New York: Grune & Stratton 1972.

Charkes, N.D., Dugan, M.A., Maier, W.P., Saulen, R., Escovitz, E., Learner, N., Dubin, R., Kazar, J.: Scintigraphic detection of deep-vein thrombosis with ^{131}I-fibrinogen. J. nucl. Med. **15**, 1163–1166 (1974).

Chervu, L.R., Freeman, L.M., Blaufox, M.D.: Radiopharmaceuticals for renal studies. Semin. nucl. Med. **4**, 3–22 (1974).

Cho, S.I., Derhagopian, R.P., Krane, R.S., Libertino, J.A.: Vascular injury of cadaver kidney—detection with Xenon-133 technique. Urology **3**, 15–17 (1974).

Coe, F.L., Burke, G.: A theoretical approach to the I^{131} Hippuran renogram. J. nucl. Med. **5**, 555–561 (1964).

Cohen, M.L.: Radionuclide clearance techniques. Semin. nucl. Med. **4**, 23–38 (1974).

Concannon, J.P., Summers, R.E., Brewer, R., Cole, C., Weil, C., Foster, W.D.: I^{125} Allyl inulin for the determination of glomerular filtration rate. Amer. J. Roentgenol. **92**, 302–308 (1964).

Constable, A.R., Joekes, A.M.: Scintigraphy with renography applied to the duplex kidney. In: Radionuclides in Nephrology (Blaufox, M.D. and Funck-Bretano, J.-L., eds.), pp. 267–272. New York: Grune & Stratton 1972.

Conway, J.J.: Considerations for the performance of radionuclide procedures in children. Semin. nucl. Med. **2**, 305–315 (1972).

Conway, J.J., Belman, A.B., King, L.R.: Direct and indirect radionuclide cystography. Semin. nucl. Med. **4**, 197–211 (1974).

Corriere, J.N., Jr., Kuhl, D.E., Murphy, J.J.: The use of ^{99m}Tc labeled sulfur colloid to study particle dynamics in the urinary tract: vesicoureteral reflux. Invest. Urol. **4**, 570 (1967).

Cosgrove, M.D., Evans, K., Raphael, M.J.: The use of Xenon-133 to measure renal blood flow in patients. Brit. J. Surg. **55**, 245–249 (1968).

Cosgrove, M.D., Mowat, P.: Evaluation of the Xenon-133 renal blood flow method. Brit. J. Urol. **46**, 134–147 (1974).

Crandell, D.C., Friedman, B.I., Britt, L.G., Booth, A.S., Jr.: Scintillation camera imaging of post-renal transplantation ureteral death. Radiology **102**, 663–664 (1972).

Current Aspects of Nuclear Medicine. J. Wadsworth Hospital. **14** (2), 1–47 (1972).

Dabaj, E., Menges, H., Pritchard, W.H.: Determination of renal blood flow by single injection of Hippuran-I^{131} in man. Amer. Heart J. **71**, 79–83 (1966).

Davies, E.R.: Topographical scintigraphy of the kidney. Brit. med. Bull. **28**, 205–209 (1972).

Dayton, D.A., Maher, F.T., Elveback, L.R.: Renal clearance of technetium (^{99m}Tc) as pertechnetate. Mayo Clin. Proc. **44**, 549–551 (1969).

DiOrio, V.J., Jr., Mishkin, F.S.: Renal Scanning for detection of renovascular hypertension. Amer. J. Roentgenol. **109**, 769–775 (1970).

Ditzel, J., Vestergaard, P., Brinklov, M.: Glomerular filtration rate determined by ^{51}Cr-EDTA-complex. Scand. J. Urol. Nephrol. **6**, 166–170 (1972).

Donadio, J.V., Farmer, Ch.D., Hunt, J.C., Tauxe, W.N., Hallenbeck, G.A., Shorter, R.G.: Renal function in donors and recipients of renal allotransplantation: radioisotopic measurements. Ann. intern. Med. **66**, 105–115 (1967).

Donath, A.: The simultaneous determination in children of glomerular filtration rate and effective renal plasma flow by the single injection clearance technique. Acta paediat. scand. **60**, 512–520 (1971).

Dore, E.K., Taplin, G.V., Johnson, D.E., Cockett, A.T.: Quantitative radiorenography in the diagnosis of renal hypertension. J. Urol. (Baltimore) **95**, 670–677 (1966).

Dubois, D., Nouel, J.P., Fillastre, J.P.: A scintiscan study of renal form and function using Technetium-labeled ferrous ascorbate. J. Urol. (Baltimore) **108**, 843–845 (1972).

Eckelman, W.C., Reba, R.C., Kubota, H., Stevenson, J.S.: ^{99m}Tc-Pyrophosphate for bone imaging. J. nucl. Med. **15**, 279–283 (1974).

Egleston, T.A., Acchiardo, S., Rodriguez-Antunez, A., Nakamoto, S.: ^{131}I Hippuran in the evaluation of transplanted kidneys. Radiology **93**, 1145–1148 (1969).

Elwood, Ch.M., Armenia, J., Orman, D., Morris, A., Sigman, E.: Measurement of renal plasma flow by Iodopyracet-I^{131}. J. Amer. med. Ass. **193**, 771–774 (1965).

Elwood, Ch.M., Sigman, E.M.: The measurement of merular filtration rate and effective renal plasma flow in man by Iothalamate ^{125}I and Iodopyracet ^{131}I. Circulation **36**, 441–448 (1967).

Evans, B.B., Bueschen, A.J., Colfry, A.J., Jr., Schlegel, J.U.: ^{131}I Hippuran quantitative scintillation camera studies in the evaluation and management of vesicoureteral reflux. Trans. Amer. Ass. gen. urin. Surg. **66**, 89–93 (1974).

Farmelant, M.H., Burrows, B.A.: The renogram: Physiologic basis and current clinical use. Semin. nucl. Med. **4**, 61–73 (1974).

Farmelant, M.H., Sachs, Ch.E., Burrows, B.A.: The influence of tissue background radioactivity on the apparent renal accumulation of radioactive compounds. J. nucl. Med. **11**, 112–117 (1970).

Farmelant, M.H., Sachs, Ch.E., Genna, S., Burrows, B.A.: A physiological model for the renal excretion of labeled compounds. J. nucl. Med. **10**, 664–671 (1969).

Figueroa, J.E.: The renogram and renal scintigram in clinical medicine. Sth. med. J. (Bgham, Ala.) **63**, 129–134 (1970).

Figueroa, J.E., Maxfield, W.S., Batson, H.M., Birchall, Jr., R.: Radioisotope renal function studies in human renal allografts: value in the differential diagnosis of oliguria in the presence of obstructive disease with and without urinary extravasation. J. Urol. (Baltimore) **100**, 104–108 (1968a).

Figueroa, J.E., Maxfield, W.S., Batson, H.M., Jr., Birchall, R.: Radioisotope renography and scintiscanning in renal transplantation: experience with 12 patients. Sth. med. J. (Bgham, Ala.) **61**, 565–570 (1968b).

Figueroa, J., Rodriguez-Antunez, A., Nakamoto, S., Dolff, W.J.: The scintigram after renal transplantation in man. New Engl. J. Med. **273**, 1406–1410 (1965).

Fitzer, P.M.: ^{99m}Tc-Polyphosphate Concentration in a Neuroblastoma. J. nucl. Med. **15**, 904–906 (1974).

Fletcher, J.W., Butler, R.L., Henry, R.E., Solaric-George, E., Donati, R.M.: Bone marrow scanning in Paget's disease. JNM/Concise Communication **14**, 928–930 (1973).

Fletcher, J.W., Solaric-George, E., Henry, R.E., Donati, R.M.: Evaluation of ^{99m}Tc-pyrophosphate as a bone imaging agent. Radiology **109**, 467–469 (1973).

Forman, B.H., Antar, M.A., Touloukian, R.J., Mulrow, P.J., Genel, M.: Localization of a metastatic adrenal carcinoma using ^{131}I-19-iodocholesterol. J. nucl. Med. **15**, 332–334 (1974).

Fozzard, H.A.: Diodrast (I^{131}) whole blood clearance as an index of renal blood flow. Amer. J. Physiol. **206**, 309–312 (1964).

Frankel, R.S., Jones, A.E., Johnson, K.W., Johnston, G.S.: The significance of urinary bladder displacement noted on whole-body ^{18}F bone scintigraphy. Radiology **109**, 397–399 (1973).

Freedman, G.S.: Radionuclide imaging of the injured patient. Radiol. Clin. N. Amer. **11**, 461–477 (1973).

Freedman, G.S., Goodwin, P.N., Johnson, Ph.M., Pierson, R.N.: An evaluation of the image-intensifier scintillation camera with some comparisons to the single crystal camera. Radiology **92**, 21–29 (1969).

Freedman, G.S., Schiff, M., Jr., Lange, R.C., Brown, R.S., Weiss, R.M., Treves, S., Lytton, B.: Functional assessment of renal homografts by means of ^{99m}Tc-DTPA and a gamma scintillation camera. Invest. Urol. **9**, 490–495 (1972).

Freeman, L.M.: Rapid blood flow scintiphotographic studies of renal trauma and infarction. In: Radionuclides in Nephrology (Blaufox, M.D. and Funck-Bretano, J.-L., eds.), pp. 281–287. New York: Grune & Stratton 1972.

Freeman, L.M.: Scintigraphy in diseases of the urinary tract. A. renal cysts and tumors. In: Progress in nuclear medicine, Chapter 13, Volume 2 (Blaufox, M.D., ed.), pp. 274–282. Baltimore: University Park Press 1972.

Freeman, L.M.: Scintigraphy in diseases of the urinary tract: B. Renal infarction. In: Progress in Nuclear Medicine, Chapter 13, Volume 2 (Blaufox, M.D., ed.). Baltimore: University Park Press 1972.

Freeman, L.M., Meng, C.-H., Bernstein, R.G., Blaufox, M.D.: Rapid, sequential renal blood flow scintiphotography. Radiology **92**, 918–923 (1969).

Freeman, L.M., Meng, C.-H., Richter, M.W., Blaufox, M.D.: Patency of major renal vascular pathways demonstrated by rapid blood flow scintiphotography. J. Urol. (Baltimore) **105**, 473–481 (1971).

Freeman, L.M., Goldman, S.M., Shaw, R.K., Blaufox, M.D.: Kidney visualization with ^{131}I-ortho-iodohippurate in patients with renal insufficiency. J. nucl. Med. **10**, 545–549 (1969).

Freeman, L.M., Johnson, P.M.: Renal imaging with radionuclides. In: Progress in Nuclear Medicine, Chapter 9, Volume 2 (Blaufox, M.D., ed.), pp. 163–198. Baltimore: University Park Press 1972.

Fritjofsson, A., Persson, J.E., Soderholm, B., Vikterlof, K.J.: Quantitative determination of kidney function using radiorenography. Scand. J. Urol. Nephrol **7**, 215–222 (1973).

Fusco, M.A., Peek, N.F., Jungerman, J.A., Zielinski, F.W., deNardo, S.J., deNardo, G.L.: Production of carrier-free ^{123}I using the ^{127}I (p, 5n) ^{123}Xe reaction. J. nucl. Med. **13**, 729–732 (1972).

Gagnon, J.A., Mailloux, L.U., Doolittle, J.E., Teschan, P.E.: An isotopic method for instantaneous measurements of effective renal blood flow. Amer. J. Physiol. **218**, 180–186 (1970).

Gedgaudas, E., White, R.I., Jr., Loken, M.K.: Radiology in renal transplantation. Radiol. Clin. N. Amer. **10**, 529–544 (1972).

Gilday, D.L., Alderson, Ph.O.: Scintigraphic evaluation of liver and spleen injury. Semin. nucl. Med. **4**, 357–409 (1974).

Goergen, Th.G., Alazraki, N.P., Halpern, S.E., Heath, V., Ashburn, W.L.: "Cold" bone lesions: a newly recognized phenomenon of bone imaging. J. nucl. Med. **15**, 1120–1124 (1974).

Goluboff, B., Bogash, M., Cope, C., Wolgin, W., Isard, H.J.: Renal blood flow measured by radioxenon 133: evaluation of a technique in dogs. J. appl. Physiol. **26**, 208–214 (1969).

Gotta, H., Chwojnik, A., Fedchteyn, S., Pecorini, V.: Diagnosis of vascular and nonvascular renal tumors. Differentiation with double isotope scintigraphy and radioactivity curves. J. nucl. Biol. Med. **17**, 151–157 (1973).

Gottschalk, A.: Radioisotope scintiphotography with Technetium 99m and the gamma scintillation camera. Amer. J. Roentgenol. **97**, 860–868 (1966).

Gottschalk, A., Anger, H.O.: Use of the scintillation camera to reduce radioisotope scanning time. J. Amer. med. Ass. **192**, 448–452 (1965).

Grove, R.B., Reba, R.C., Eckelman, W.C., Goodyear, M.: Clinical evaluation of radiolabeled Bleomycin (BLEO) for tumor detection. J. nucl. Med. **15**, 386–390 (1974).

Grunfeld, J.P., Sabto, J., Bankir, L., Funck-Bretano, J.-L.: Methods for measurement of renal blood flow in man. Semin. nucl. Med. **4**, 39–49 (1974).

Gussin, R.Z., Cafruny, E.J.: Effects of ethacrynic acid on renal uptake of mercury. J. Pharmacol. exp. Ther. **149**, 1–6 (1965).

Halko, A., Burke, G., Sorkin, A., Enenstein, J.: Computer-aided statistical analysis of the scintillation camera ^{131}I-Hippuran renogram. J. nucl. Med. **14**, 253–264 (1973).

Hallwachs, O., zum Winkel, K., Steinhausen, M., Rohl, L.: Radioisotopes used to determine tubular passage time in dog kidneys. Scand. J. Urol. Nephrol. **4**, 248–251 (1970).

Hallwachs, O., Ziegler, M., Winkel, K. zum: Radioisotopenverfahren, seitengetrennte Nierenfunktionsprüfungen und Angiotensininfusionstest bei Hochdruckkranken mit Nierenarterienstenosen. Urologe **1**, 22–32 (1967).

Halpern, S., Tubis, M., Endow, J., Walsh, C., Kunsa, J., Zwicker, B.: ^{99m}Tc-Penicillamine-acetazolamide complex: A new renal scanning agent. J. nucl. Med. **13**, 45–50 (1972).

Halpern, S.W., Tubis, M., Golden, M., Kunsa, J., Endow, J., Walsh, C.: ^{99m}TPAC, a new renal scanning agent: II. Evaluation in humans. J. nucl. Med. **13**, 723–728 (1972).

Harbert, J.C., Ashburn, W.L., Davidson, J.D.: An improved method of renography using the split crystal scintillation camera. J. Urol. (Baltimore) **90**, 681–687 (1968).

Harbert, J.C., Fraley, E.E., Deckers, P.J.: Alterations in radioactive isotope renogram pattern with urinary bladder filling. J. Amer. med. Ass. **211**, 810–811 (1970).

Harries, J.D., Mildenberger, R.R., Malowany, A.S., Drummond, K.N.: A computerized cumulative integral method for the precise measurement of the glomerular filtration rate. Proc. Soc. exp. Biol. (N.Y.) **140**, 1148–1155 (1972).

Hartenbower, D.L., Winston, M.A., Weiss, E.R., Coburn, J.W.: The scintillation camera in embolic acute renal failure. J. Urol. (Baltimore) **104**, 799–802 (1970).

Hayes, M.: Early detection and classification of renal transplant rejection by B/K scan ratio and blood isotope clearance data. Transplantation **12**, 139–141 (1971).

Hayes, M., Moore, Th.C., Taplin, G.V.: Radionuclide procedures in predicting early renal transplant rejection. Radiology **103**, 627–631 (1972).

Haynie, Th., Stewart, B.H., Nofal, M.M., Carr, E.A., Jr., Beierwaltes, W.H.: Diagnosis of renal vascular disease and renal tumors by photoscanning. J. Amer. med. Ass. **179**, 137–140 (1962).

Haynie, Th.P., Stewart, B.H., Nofal, M.M., Carr, E.A., Beierwaltes, W.H.: Renal scintiscans in the diagnosis of renal vascular disease. J. nucl. Med. **2**, 272–281 (1961).

Hegesippe, M., Beydon, J., Bardy, A., Panneciere, C.: Stannous pyrophosphate labeled with Technetium-99m for skeletal scintigraphy. J. nucl. Biol. Med. **17**, (3), 93–96 (1973).

Heiskanen, T.Weber, Grasbeck, R.: Determination of ^{131}I-hippuric acid renal clearance, using single injection techniques. Scand. J. clin. Lab. Invest. **21**, 211–215 (1968).

Henk, J.M., Cottrall, M.F., Taylor, D.M.: Radiation dosimetry of the I-Hippuran renogram. Brit. J. Radiol. **4**, 327–334 (1967).

Hertsch, G.J., Melton, M.L., Mooney, R.T.: A TV system for data blending and contrast enhancement of scintiscans. Amer. J. Roentgenol. **106**, 871–873 (1969).

Herwig, K.R., Conn, J.W., Schteingart, D.E., Beierwaltes, W.H.: Localization of adrenal tumors by photoscanning. J. Urol. (Baltimore) **109**, 2–4 (1973).

Hirakawa, A., Kuwahara, M., Ueyama, H.: Analog computer-aided RI renogram diagnosis. In: Radionuclides in Nephrology (Blaufox, M.D. and Funck-Bretano, J.-L., eds.), pp. 303–314. New York: Grune & Stratton 1972.

Hiramatsu, Y., O'Mara, R.E., McAfee, J.G., Markarian, B.: Intrarenal distribution of diagnostic agents. Invest. Radiol. **5**, 295–310 (1970).

Hisada, K., Ando, A.: Radiolanthanides as promising tumor scanning agents. J. nucl. Med. **14**, 615–617 (1973).

Hisada, K., Tonami, N., Hiraki, T., Ando, A.: Tumor scanning with ^{169}Yb-citrate. J. nucl. Med. **15**, 210–212 (1974).

Hodson, C.J.: Physiological changes in size of the human kidney. Clin. Radiol. **12**, 91 (1961).

Hoffer, P.B., Lathrop, K., Bekerman, C., Fang, V.S., Refetoff, S.: "Preprint." Use of ^{131}I-CEA antibody as a tumor scanning agent. Personal Communication.

Hoffer, P.B., Oppenheim, B.E., Sterling, M.L., Yasillo, N.: A simple device for reducing motion artifacts in Gamma camera images. Radiology **103**, 199–200 (1972).

Hollenberg, N.K.: Renal blood flow in hypertension and in renal disease. In: Progress in Nuclear Medicine, Chapter 10, Volume 2 (Blaufox, M.D., ed.), pp. 138–142. Baltimore: University Park Press 1972.

Hollenberg, N.D., Adams, D.F., Abrams, H.L., Merrill, J.P.: The relationship between intrarenal perfusion and sodium homeostasis in man. In: Radionuclides in Nephrology (Blaufox, M.D. and Funck-Bretano, J.-L., eds.), pp. 37–46. New York: Grune & Stratton 1972.

Hor, G.: Advantages and limitations of radioisotope clearance methods from a clinician's point of view. J. nucl. Biol. Med. **16**, 167–176 (1972).

Horst, W., Rosler, H., Schneider, C., Conrad, B.: Radio-nephrography and renal scintigram: combined investigation of renal function and structure. Germ. med. Monthly **7**, 186–188 (1962).

Hurwitz, S.R., Ashburn, W.L., Green, J.P., Halpern, S.E.: Clinical applications of a "portable" scintillation camera. J. nucl. Med. **14**, 585–587 (1973).

Inasaka, T.: Studies of the intrarenal distribution of blood flow with ^{133}Xe in diseased human kidney. Jap. Circulat. J. 737–748 (1969).
Izenstark, J.L., Burden, J.J., Mardis, H.K., Varela, R.: Clinical indications for kidney scanning. J. Amer. med. Ass. **188**, 136–139 (1964).
Jackman, S.J., Maher, F.T., Hattery, R.R.: Detection of renal-cell carcinoma with ^{99m}Tc polyphosphate imaging of bone. A case report. Mayo Clin. Proc. **49**, 297–299 (1974).
Jeremy, D., Melver, M.: Inulin, ^{57}Co-labelled vitamin B_{12} and endogenous creatinine clearances in the measurement of glomerular filtration rate in man. Aust. Ann. Med. **15**, 346–351 (1966).
Joekes, A.M.: Isotopes and the kidney. Brit. med. Bull. **28**, 200–204 (1972).
Joekes, A.M.: Obstructive uropathy. Semin. nucl. Med. **4**, 187–196 (1974).
Johnson, A.E., Gollan, F.: Determination of glomerular filtration rate by external monitoring of Chromium-51 labeled inulin. Int. J. appl. Radiat. **19**, 43–47 (1968).
Johnston, G.S., Murphy, G.P.: The effect of acute and chronic ureteral occlusions upon renal handling of Hg^{203} Chlomerodrin. Amer. J. Roentgenol. **98**, 162–171 (1966).
Kahn, R.J., Gottingnies, P., Venherweghem, J.L., Lambert, P.P.: Control experiments on the measurement of the renal blood flow by the Xenon 133 washout technique. In: Radionuclides in Nephrology (Blaufox, M.D. and Funck-Bretano, J.-L., eds.), pp. 99–103. New York: Grune & Stratton 1972.
Kaplan, W., Holman, B.L., Liebow, P.A., Davis, M.A.: Enhanced detection of a skeletal lesion with delayed ^{99m}Tc-polyphosphate bone scanning. J. nucl. Med. **15**, 47–49 (1974).
Katul, M.J., Wax, S.H.: Evaluation of renal function during experimental hydronephrosis by means of the radioisotope renogram. Surg. Gynec. Obstet. **126**, 363–371 (1968).
Keane, J.M., Schlegel, J.U.: The use of a scintillation camera system for screening of hypertensive patients. J. Urol. (Baltimore) **108**, 12–14 (1972).
Kereiakes, J.G., Wellman, H.M., Simmons, G., Saenger, E.L.: Radiopharmaceutical dosimetry in pediatrics. Semin. nucl. Med. **2**, 316–327 (1972).
Kessler, R.H., Weinstein, S.W., Nash, F.D., Fujimoto, M.: Effects of chlormerodrin, p-chloromercuibenzoate and dichlorophenamide on renal sodium reabsorption and oxygen consumption. Nephron **1**, 221–229 (1964).
Keyes, J.W., Gazella, G.R., Strange, D.R.: Image analysis by one line minicomputer for improved camera quality control. J. nucl. Med. **13**, 525–527 (1972).
The kidney. In: Physicians' Desk Reference for Radiology and Nuclear Medicine (Blaufox, M.D. and Freeman, L.N., Editorial Consultants), pp. 58–62. Oradell, N.J.: Medical Economics Company 1973.
Kirsch, W., May, P., Oberhausen, E.: Determination of the split effective renal plasma flow with ^{131}I Hippuran, an experimental and clinical study. Urologe **9**, 135–139 (1970).
Kiviat, M.D., Griep, R.J.: Pyelonephrosis complicating ureteral obstruction: a limitation of renal scintiscanning in predicting reversibility of renal damage. J. Urol. (Baltimore) **109**, 339–341 (1973).
Klopper, J.F., Hauser, W., Atkins, H.L., Eckelman, W.C., Richards, P.: Evaluation of ^{99m}Tc-DTPA for the measurement of glomerular filtration rate. J. nucl. Med. **12**, 107–110 (1972).
Koenigsberg, M., Blaufox, M.D., Freeman, L.M.: Traumatic injuries of the renal vasculature and parenchyma. Semin. nucl. Med. **4**, 117–132 (1974).
Komorn, R., Cafruny, E.J.: Effects of ethacrynic acid on renal protein-bound sulfhydryl groups. J. Pharmacol. exp. Ther. **148**, 367–372 (1965).
Koss, L.G., Melamed, M.R., Ricci, A., Melock, W.F., Kelly, R.E.: Carcinogenesis in the human urinary bladder: Observations after exposure to para-amino diphenyl. New Engl. J. Med. **272**, 767 (1965).
Kountz, S.: Radionuclides and renal transplantation. In: Progress in Nuclear Medicine, Chapter 11, Volume 2 (Blaufox, M.D., ed.), pp. 235–248. Baltimore: University Park Press 1972.

Kountz, S.L., Yeh, S.H., Wood, J., Cohn, R., Kriss, J.P.: Technetium-99m(v)-citrate complex for estimation of glomerular filtration rate. Nature (Lond.) **215**, 1397–1399 (1967).
Kriss, J.P.: Radioisotope scanning in medical diagnosis. Ann. Rev. Med. **14**, 381–406 (1963).
Laakso, L., Lindgren, I., Rekonen, A.: Radiomercury and rat kidney. Excerpta Acta radiol. **3**, 305–309 (1965).
Ladefoged, J., Petersen, F.: Hemodynamic studies in acute renal failure. In: Radionuclides in Nephrology (Blaufox, M.D. and Funck-Bretano, J.-L., eds.), pp. 47–54. New York: Grune & Stratton 1972.
Lambrecht, R.M., Norton, E., Wolf, A.P.: Kit for carrier-free ^{123}I sodium iodide, 8. J. nucl. Med. **14**, 269–273 (1973).
Langhammer, H., Galubit, G., Grebe, S.F., Hampe, J.F., Haubold, U., Hor, G., Kaul, A., Koeppe, P., Koppenhagen, J., Roedler, H.D., van der Schoot, J.B.: ^{67}Ga for tumor scanning. J. nucl. Med. **13**, 25–30 (1972).
Lavender, S.: Estimation of glomerular filtration rate and effective renal plasma flow by isotopic methods. Brit. J. Urol., Suppl., 76–89 (1969).
Lawrence, D., Mishkin, F.: Radionuclide imaging in epididymo-orchitis. J. Urol. (Baltimore) **112**, 387–389 (1974).
Lentle, B.C., Castor, W.R., Brown, L.B., Glazebrook, B.A.: Renography in the diagnosis of obstructive uropathy due to malignant tumors of the pelvis. Surg. Gynec. Obstet. **139**, 353–354 (1974).
Lerson, G., Delwaide, P.A., Lejeune, G., Rorive, G., Merchie, G.: The value of two simplified methods for the measurement of renal plasma flow by ^{131}I Hippuran. In: Radionuclides in Nephrology (Blaufox, M.D. and Funck-Bretano, J.-L., eds.), pp. 241–248. New York: Grune & Stratton 1972.
Lewis, D.H., Bergentz, S.E.: Renal blood flow measurement with Xenon-133 at the time of operation for renal artery stenosis. Surgery **59**, 1043–1049 (1966).
Lewis, D.H., Bergentz, S.E., Brunius, U., Ekman, H., Gelin, L.E.: Value of renal blood flow measurement with Xenon-133 at the time of kidney transplants. Ann. Surg. **166**, 67–74 (1967).
Lewis, D.H., Bergentz, S.E., Brunius, U., Ekman, H., Gelin, L.E., Hood, B.: Blood flow in kidney transplants: A clinical evaluation of the ^{133}Xenon method. Scand. J. Urol. Nephrol. **2**, 36–39 (1968).
Lewis, D.H., Fritjofsson, A.: Comparison of Xenon-133 washout curves from the kidney with direct measurement of renal venous outflow. Scand. J. Urol. Nephrol. **2**, 62–63 (1968).
Lingardh, G.: Separate renal function in man determined by a combined procedure using a dye-dilution method and radioisotopes. Scand. J. Urol. Nephrol., reprint, 1971, pp. 1–4.
Lingardh, G.: Studies on separate renal blood flow and function using a dye-dilution technique and radiochemicals. Scand. J. Urol. Nephrol.,Suppl. **8**, 1–29 (1971).
Linnemann, R.E., Loken, M.K., Markland, C.: Computerized compartmental renograms to study kidney function. J. Urol. (Baltimore) **103**, 533–538 (1970).
Lipshultz, L.I., Corriere, J.N.: Dual isotope scintiscan: new method for evaluating bladder function. Urology **4**, 267–270 (1974).
Loken, M.K., Linnemann, R.E., Kush, G.S.: Evaluation of renal function using a scintillation camera and computer. Radiology **93**, 85–94 (1969).
Lubin, E., Levitus, Z., Shimeoni, A.: Rapid sequential kidney scanning with ^{131}I-Hippuran. J. nucl. Med. **9**, 567–570 (1968).
Lucey, D.T., Smith, M.J.V.: Initial diagnosis and management of urinary tract injuries. Clin. Med. **80**, 17–26 (1973).
Lundgren, G., Ekman, L., Hansson, E., Magnusson, G., Nordstrom, M.: Renographic and autoradiographic studies during rejection in canine renal allografts. Acta chir. scand., Suppl. 382 (1967).

Lutzker, L., Koenigsberg, M., Meng, C.-H., Greeman, L.M.: The role of radionuclide imaging in spleen trauma. Radiology **110**, 419–425 (1973).

Mac Ewan, D.W., Rosenthall, L.: Assessment of excretory urography and radioisotope renal scanning in diseases of the kidneys. Radiology **86**, 1010–1020 (1966).

Magnusson, G.: Quantitative ^{131}I Hippuran renography. Critical aspects based on studies of the extrarenal component of the renogram in bilaterally nephrectomized patients. In: Radionuclides in Nephrology (Blaufox, M.D. and Funck-Bretano, J.-L., eds.), pp. 325–332. New York: Grune & Stratton 1972.

Maher, F.T., Elveback, L.: Simultaneous renal clearances of ^{125}I and ^{131}I-labelled orthoiodohippurate and para-aminohippurate in the estimation of effective renal plasma flow in man. Mayo Clin. Proc. **45**, 657–661 (1970).

Maher, F.T., Tauxe, W.N.: Renal clearance in man of pharmaceuticals containing radioactive iodine. J. Amer. med. Ass. **207**, 97–104 (1969).

Mailloux, L., Gagnon, J.A.: Measurement of effective renal plasma flow. In: Progress in Nuclear Medicine, Chapter 4, Volume 2 (Blaufox, M.D., ed.), pp. 54–70. Baltimore: University Park Press 1972.

Mandel, P., Saxe, B., Spatz, M.: Urologic serendipity in whole body bone scanning. Urology **3**, 283–287 (1974).

Martin, D.C., Hunter, J.L., Lawton, M.B., Berke, R.A., Morton, N.E.: Serial radionuclide quantitative function studies for evaluation of renal transplants. J. Urol. (Baltimore) **112**, 2–6 (1974).

Mason, D.T., Ashburn, W.L., Harbert, J.C., Cohen, L.S., Braunwalk, E.: Rapid sequential visualization of the heart and great vessels in man using the wide-field anger scintillation camera. Circulation **39**, 19–28 (1969).

Maxwell, M.H., Hayes, M.: The abnormal renogram: A. The renogram in hypertension. In: Progress in Nuclear Medicine, Chapter 12, Volume 2 (Blaufox, M.D., ed.), pp. 249–259. Baltimore: University Park Press 1972.

McAfee, J.G., Reba, R.C., Chodos, R.B.: Radioisotopic methods in the transplanted kidney as a signal of rejection. Surgery **58**, 815–818 (1965).

McCready, V.R.: Clinical radioisotope scanning. J. Radiol. **40**, 401–423 (1967).

McCready, V.R., Bentley, R.F., Popham, M.G.: The use of a gamma camera computer link for long-term dynamic studies on the kidney. In: Radionuclides in Nephrology (Blaufox, M.D. and Funck-Bretano, J.-L., eds.), pp. 251–256. New York: Grune & Stratton 1972.

McKeighen, R.E., Muehllehner, G., Moyer, R.A.: Gamma camera collimator considerations for imaging ^{123}I. J. nucl. Med. **15**, 328–331 (1974).

McNeil, B.J., Holman, B.L., Adelstein, S.J.: The scintigraphic definition of pulmonary embolism. J. Amer. med. Ass. **227**, 753–756 (1974).

Meier, D.A., Beierwaltes, W.H.: Radioisotope renal studies and renal hypertension. J. Amer. med. Ass. **198**, 1257–1262 (1966).

Meldolesi, U., Mombelli, L., Roncari, G., Conte, L.: A simple method of estimating renal clearance by renography. J. nucl. Biol. Med. **17**, 79–83 (1973).

Meschan, I., Watts, F.C., Lathem, E., Boyce, W.H., Schmid, H.E., Maynard, C.D., Roper, T., Hosnick, T.A.: Simultaneous PAH, inulin, and Renografin-I^{131} renal clearance determinations and a method for calculating Renografin clearance from renograms in patients. Amer. J. Roentgenol. **97**, 909–919 (1966).

Meschan, I., Watts, F.C., Maynard, C.D., Schultz, J.L., Bolliger, T.T., Morris, M.L.: The quantitation of the Renografin-Iodine-131 renogram for renal clearance determination. J. nucl. Med. **7**, 442–453 (1966).

Meschan, I., Watts, F.C., Maynard, C.D., Witcofski, R.L., Smith, S.N.: Quantification of the glomerular filtration of the individual kidney by the I^{131} Renografin renogram. Radiology **88**, 984–987 (1967).

Miller, St.W., Castronovo, F.P., Pendergrass, H.P., Potsaid, M.S.: Technetium 99m labeled diphosphonate bone scanning in Paget's disease. Amer. J. Roentgenol. **121**, 177–183 (1974).

Milstein, D.M., Lee, H.B., Liang, Th., Blaufox, M.D.: Glomerular blood flow distribution in the rat: Preliminary observations. In: Radionuclides in Nephrology (Blaufox, M.D. and Funck-Bretano, J.-L., eds.), pp. 14–20. New York: Grune & Stratton 1972.

Mobley, J.E., Schlegel, J.U.: Radiohippuran accumulation in the transplanted kidney as a signal of rejection. Surgery **58**, 815–818 (1965).

Mogensen, P., Rossing, N., Giese, J.: Glomerular filtration rate measurement and ^{131}I-Hippuran renography before unilateral nephrectomy. Scand. J. Urol. Nephrol. **6**, 228–231 (1972).

Morales, J.O.: Space-occupying Lesions of the Kidney. Semin. nucl. Med. **4**, 133–149 (1974).

Morales, J.O., Goldberg, B.B.: Telephone transmission of scintiphotographs. J. nucl. Med. **13**, 771–772 (1972).

Morehouse, D.D., Belitsky, Ph., Mackinnon, K.: Rupture of the posterior urethra. J. Urol. (Baltimore) **107**, 255–258 (1972).

Morel, F.: Criticism of the techniques available for measuring medullary renal blood flow. In: Radionuclides in Nephrology (Blaufox, M.D. and Funck-Bretano, J.-L., eds.), pp. 93–98. New York: Grune & Stratton 1972.

Morris, A.M., Elwood, Ch., Sigman, E.M., Catanzaro, A.: The renal clearance of ^{131}I labeled meglumine diatrizoate (Renografin) in man. J. nucl. Med. **6**, 183–191 (1965).

Mosbaugh, Ph.G.: Testicular scanning. Urologists' Correspondence Club, 1974.

Murphy, G.P., Schirmer, H.K.A., Johnston, G.S., Morris, R.A.: Clinical correlations of Hg^{203} Chlormerodrin and urinary concentration in hypertension and renal disease. J. Urol. (Baltimore) **98**, 163–166 (1967).

Nebesar, R.A., Rabinov, K.R., Potsaid, M.S.: Radionuclide imaging of the spleen in suspected splenic injury. Radiology **110**, 609–614 (1974).

Nebesar, R.A., Tefft, M., Feller, R.M.: Correlation of angiography and isotope scanning in abdominal diseases of children. Amer. J. Roentgenol. **109**, 323–340 (1970).

Norman, N.: Effective plasma flow of the individual kidney: determination on the basis of the (^{131}I) Hippuran renogram. Scand. J. clin. Lab. Invest. **30**, 395–403 (1972).

O'Dell, R.M.: Determination of glomerular filtration rate by use of single injection of Iodine-131 labelled sodium diatrizoate. J. nucl. Med. **7**, 470–472 (1966).

Oeser, H., Billion, H.: Funktionelle Strahlendiagnostik durch etikettierte Röntgenkonstrastmittel. Fortschr. Röntgenstr. **76**, 431 (1952).

Oester, A., Wolf, H., Madsen, P.O.: Double isotope technique in renal function testing in dogs. Invest. Urol. **6**, 387–392 (1969).

Olbing, H., Strotges, M.W., Strohmenger, P.: Examination of vesicoureteral reflux with Iodine 125: significance for the decision of treatment. In: Radionuclides in Nephrology (Blaufox, M.D. and Funck-Bretano, J.-L., eds.), pp. 295–300. New York: Grune & Stratton 1972.

O'Neill, J.A., Maxfield, W.S.: ^{131}I camera renogram for detection of urologic pathology in the newborn. J. pediat. Surg. **7**, 236–242 (1972).

Pavel, D.: Some aspects of radioisotope scintiscanning in normal and pathologic kidney. Rev. roum. Med. interne **5**, 265–281 (1968).

Pavel, D., Chanard, J.: Renography in patients with acute renal failure in the polyuric stage. In: Radionuclides in Nephrology (Blaufox, M.D. and Funck-Bretano, J.-L., eds.), pp. 351–360. New York: Grune & Stratton 1972.

Pedersen, F., Ladefoged, J.: Renal hemodynamics in acute renal failure in man measured by intra-arterial injection: external counting techniques with Xenon-133 and I-131-Albumin. Scand. J. Urol. Nephrol. **7**, 187–195 (1973).

Pedersen, J.F., Madsen, P.O.: Simultaneous determination of glomerular filtration rate and effective plasma flow by external monitoring of radioisotopes: an experimental study in dogs. Invest. Urol. **8**, 203–209 (1970).

Peters, P.E., Ter-Pogossian, M.M., Rockoff, M.L., Metzger, J.M., Koehler, P.R.: Measurement of renal blood flow by means of radioactive water labeled with Oxygen 15. In: Radionuclides in Nephrology (Blaufox, M.D. and Funck-Bretano, J.-L., eds.), pp. 27–36. New York: Grune & Stratton 1972.

Pinter, G.G.: Adequacy and limitations of the semiconductor radiation detector technique in measuring blood flow distribution in renal tissue. In: Radionuclides in Nephrology (Blaufox, M.D. and Funck-Bretano, J.-L., eds.), pp. 23–26. New York: Grune & Stratton 1972.

Pollack, H.M., Edell, St., Morales, J.O.: Radionuclide imaging in renal pseudotumors. Radiology **111**, 639–644 (1974).

Pritchard, W.H., Eckstein, R.W., McIntyre, W.J., Dabaj, E.: Correlation of renal blood flow determined by the single-injection of Hippuran-I-131 with direct measurements of flow. Amer. Heart J. **70**, 789–796 (1965).

Quinn, J.L., Maynard, C.D.: Renal radioisotope scintiscanning. In: Radiologic Clinics of North America, Volume 3, No. 1, pp. 65–74. Philadelphia: W.B. Saunders Co. 1965.

Radwin, H.M., Novoselsky, S.P.: The Gamma camera in pediatric urologic diagnosis. J. Urol. (Baltimore) **97**, 942–947 (1967).

Radwin, H.M., O'Dell, R.M., Schlegel, J.U.: The renal response to acute partial obstruction. J. Urol. (Baltimore) **90**, 234–246 (1963).

Radwin, H.M., Schlegel, J.U.: Effect of hemodynamics on renal pelvic pressures. Surg. Forum **13**, 489–491 (1962).

Ram, M.D., Evans, K., Chisholm, G.D.: A single injection method for measurement of effective renal plasma flow. Brit. J. Urol. **40**, 425–428 (1968).

Ram, M.D., Holroyd, M., Chisholm, G.D.: Measurement of glomerular filtration-rate using ^{131}I-Diatrizoate. Lancet **1969** , 397–399.

Raynaud, C.: A technique for the quantitative measurement of the function of each kidney. Semin. nucl. Med. **4**, 51–60 (1974).

Raynaud, C., Comar, D., Buisson, M., Kellershohn, C.: Radioactive thallium: a new agent for scans of the renal medulla. In: Radionuclides in Nephrology (Blaufox, M.D. and Funck-Bretano, J.-L., eds.), pp. 289–294. New York: Grune & Stratton 1972.

Raynaud, C., Jacquot, Ch., Freeman, L.M.: Measuring renal uptake of ^{197}Hg Cl_2 by gamma camera. Radiology **110**, 413–417 (1973).

Raynaud, C., Ricard, S., Karam, Y., Kellershohn, C.: The use of the renal uptake of ^{197}Hg as a method for testing the functional value of each kidney. J. nucl. Med. **11**, 125–133 (1970).

Razzak, M.A., Botti, R.E., McIntyre, W.J., Pritchard, W.H.: Determination of renal blood flow by external monitoring of Radiohippuran disappearance. J. Urol. (Baltimore) **100**, 209–214 (1968).

Razzak, M.A., Botti, R.E., McIntyre, W.J., Pritchard, W.H.: Consecutive determination of cardiac output and renal blood flow by external monitoring of radioactive isotopes. J. nucl. Med. **11**, 190–195 (1970).

Reba, R.C., McAfee, J.C., Wagner, H.N., Jr.: Radiomercury-labelled chlormerodrin for in vivo uptake studies and scintillation scanning of unilateral renal lesions associated with hypertension. Medicine **42**, 269–296 (1963).

Reba, R.C., Poulouse, K.R., Kirchner, P.T.: Radiolabeled chelates for visualization of kidney function and structure with emphasis on their use in renal insufficiency. Semin. nucl. Med. **4**, 151–168 (1974).

Reba, R.C., Wagner, H.N., McAfee, J.C.: Measurement of Hg^{203} Chlormerodrin accumulation by the kidneys for detection of unilateral renal disease. Radiation **79**, 134 (1962).

Reichert, J.R., Tyson, I.B.: Venophotoscintigraphy in renal transplant renograms: demonstration of an unusual complication. Radiology **111**, 219–220 (1974).

Retik, A.B., Rosen, St.M., Hollenberg, N.K., Murray, J.E., Harrison, J.H.: Intrarenal distribution of blood flow in canine renal allografts treated with immunosupressive drugs. J. Urol. (Baltimore) **101**, 482–486 (1969).

Rodriguez-Antunez, A., Gill, W.M., Egleston, Th.A.: Assessment of function in the transplanted kidney with ^{131}I Hippuran. J. Urol. (Baltimore) **103**, 574–576 (1970).

Rosen, S.M., Hollenberg, N.K., Dealy, J.B., Merrill, J.P.: Measurement of the distribution of blood flow in the human kidney using the intra-arterial injection of ^{133}Xe: relationship to function in the normal and transplanted kidney. Clin. Sci. **34**, 287–302 (1968).

Rosenthall, L.: The role of radioisotope renal scanning in the assessment of renal disease. Canad. med. Ass. J. **90**, 999–1004 (1964).

Rosenthall, L.: Ortho-iodohippurate-I-131 kidney scanning in renal failure. Radiology **78**, 298–303 (1966).

Rosenthall, L.: Radionuclide diagnosis of malignant tumors of the kidney. Amer. J. Roentgenol. **101**, 662–668 (1967).

Rosenthall, L.: The use of intravenous radiopertechnetate angiography as a screening procedure for renovascular hypertension. In: Radionuclides in Nephrology (Blaufox, M.D. and Funck-Bretano, J.-L., eds.), pp. 273–280. New York: Grune & Stratton 1972.

Rosenthall, L.: Radiotechnetium renography and serial radiohippurate imaging for screening renovascular hypertension. Semin. nucl. Med. **4**, 97–116 (1974).

Rosenthall, L.: Intravenous radionuclide angiography in the diagnosis of trauma. Semin. nucl. Med. **4**, 395–409 (1974).

Rosenthall, L., Mangel, R., Lisbona, R., Lacourciere, Y.: Diagnostic applications of radiopertechnetate and radiohippurate imaging in post-renal transplantation complications. Radiology **111**, 347–358 (1974).

Rosler, H.: A semiquantitative evaluation of renograms based on a simultaneously performed simplified slope clearance. In: Radionuclides in Nephrology (Blaufox, M.D. and Funck-Bretano, J.-L., eds.), pp. 221–231. New York: Grune & Stratton 1972.

Sakurai, T., Nakarai, K.: Diagnostic value of renal angiography in renal hypertension. Acta urol. jap. **16**, 59–66 (1970).

Salvatierro, O., Jr., Powell, M.R., Price, D.C., Kountz, S.L., Belzer, F.O.: The advantages of ^{131}I-orthoiodohippurate scintiphotography in the management of patients after renal transplantation. Ann. Surg. **180**, 336–342 (1974).

Schlegel, J.U.: GU trauma slides. Medcom Famous Teachings in Modern Medicine: Gamma Camera Screening for renal and urinary tract disease. (02141).

Schlegel, J.U.: Screening for kidney and urinary tract disease. Paper presented to the Medical Section of the Amer. Life Convention, Thursday, June 11, 1970, at the Homestead, Hot Springs, Va.

Schlegel, J.U.: Scintillation camera in diagnosis of renal and urinary tract disease. Urology **2**, 361–364 (1973).

Schlegel, J.U.: Urologic injuries. Personal Communication.

Schlegel, J.U.: Hypernephroma. Urologists' Correspondence Club, 1974

Schlegel, J.U., Bakule, P.T.: A diagnostic approach in detecting renal and urinary tract disease. J. Urol. (Baltimore) **104**, 2–10 (1970).

Schlegel, J.U., Hamway, S.A.: Individual renal plasma flow determination in 2 minutes. Trans. Amer. Ass. gen.-urin. Surg. **67**, 23–26 (1975), J. Urol. (Baltimore) **116**, 282–285 (1976).

Schlegel, J.U., Merlin, A.S.: Correlation of renal mass and renal blood flow in the diagnosis of renal hypertension. Jap. J. Urol. **57**, 935–938 (1966).

Schlegel, J.U., Merlin, A.S., Varela, R.: Use of Neohydrin in scans and roentgenograms in evaluation of renal hypertension. Sth. med. J. (Bgham, Ala.) **60**, 623–626 (1967).

Schlegel, J.U., O'Dell, R.M., Izenstark, J.L.: Importance of stop flow to kidney scans. J. nucl. Med. **4**, 320–325 (1963).

Schlegel, J.U., O'Dell, R.M., Izenstark, J.L., Cuellar, J.: A technic for kidney scanning. Sth. med. J. **55**, 471–474 (1962).

Schlegel, J.U., Smith, B.G., O'Dell, R.M.: Estimation of effective renal plasma flow using I^{131}-labeled Hippuran. J. appl. Physiol. **17**, 80–82 (1962).

Schlegel, J.U., Varela, R., Stanton, J.J.: Individual renal plasma flow determination without ureteral catheterization. J. Urol. (Baltimore) **96**, 20–23 (1966).

Schlegel, J.U., Warlick, J.T. III: Experience in urologic diagnosis using a Gamma scintillation camera system. J. Urol. (Baltimore) **108**, 15–17 (1972).

Schlegel, J.U., Warlick, J.T., Smith, O.: The effect of various pharmacologic agents on renal volume. In: Renal Pharmacology (Fisher, J.W. and Cafruny, E.J., eds.), pp. 267–285. New York: Appleton-Century-Crofts 1971.

Secker-Walker, R.H., Siegel, B.A.: The use of nuclear medicine in the diagnosis of lung disease. Radiol. Clin. N. Amer. **11**, 215–241 (1973).

Semprebene, L., Benedetti-Valentini, F., Jr., Faraglia, V., Spartera, C., Pistolese, G., Citone, G., Cinotti, G., Fiorani, P.: Radio-Hippuran renography and differential renal function tests during Trimetaphan camphor-sulfonate (Arfonad) drip in prognostic evaluation of surgical management of renovascular hypertension. In: Radionuclides in Nephrology (Blaufox, M.D. and Funck-Bretano, J.-L., eds.), pp. 361–365. New York: Grune & Stratton 1972.

Servadio, C., Nissenkorn, I., Baron, J.: Radioisotope clearance using ^{99m}Tc sulfur colloid for the detection and study of vesicoureteral reflux. J. Urol. (Baltimore) **111**, 750–754 (1974).

Shapiro, R., Doppman, J., Cobb, R., Kneisel, J.J.: Major segmental renal arterial constriction: an experimental study in the dog. Radiology **85**, 462–469 (1965).

Shearer, R.J., Constable, A.R., Girling, M., Hendry, W.F., Fergusson, J.D.: Radioisotopic bone scintigraphy with the gamma camera in the investigation of prostatic cancer. Brit. med. J. **1974** , 362–365.

Skinner, D.G.: Traumatic renal artery thrombosis: A successful thrombectomy and revascularization. Ann. Surg. **177**, 264–267 (1973).

Skripka, Ch.F., Jr., Schlegel, J.U.: Accurate determination of renal function by renal histography without collection of blood or urine. II. Correlation of the renal histogram and renal function. J. Urol. (Baltimore) **114**, 809–812 (1975).

Slotkoff, L.M., Eisner, G.M., Jose, P.A., Logan, A., Lilienfield, L.S.: Microsphere measurement of the intrarenal circulation. In: Radionuclides in Nephrology (Blaufox, M.D. and Funck-Bretano, J.-L., eds.), pp. 3–8. New York: Grune & Stratton 1972.

Smith, B.G., O'Dell, R.M., Schlegel, J.U.: A simplified method of determining effective renal plasma flow. J. Urol. (Baltimore) **87**, 106–108 (1962).

Smith, P.H.: I^{131} Hippuran renography: An evaluation with observations on technique and interpretation. Brit. J. Urol. **40**, 501–513 (1968).

Sprawls, P.: Digital-computer interpretation of radioisotope distribution patterns. J. nucl. Med. **10**, 618–620 (1969).

Staab, E.V., Hopkins, J., Patton, D.D., Hanchett, J., Stone, W.J.: The use of radionuclide studies in the prediction of function in renal failure. Radiology **106**, 141–146 (1973).

Staab, E.V., Kelly, W.D., Loken, M.K.: Prognostic value of radioisotopic renograms in kidney transplantation. J. nucl. Med. **10**, 133–135 (1969).

Steinhausen, M. von, zum Winkel, K., Hallwachs, O., Ross, H.J.: Lissamin green. Glomerulare Filtration und tabulare Sekretion von J^{131} und J^{125}-Inulin bzw. J^{131}- und J^{125}-Hippuran am Hund unter Berücksichtigung auf lichtmikroskopisch bestimmte Passagezeiten von Lissamingrün. Physiologisches Institut, Strahlenklinik und Urologische Abteilung der Chirurgischen Univ. Klinik, Heidelberg. Pflügers Arch. ges. Physiol. **295**, R 57 (1967).

Stokes, J.M., Ter-Pogossian, M.: Double Isotope technique to measure renal functions. J. Amer. med. Ass. **187**, 20–23 (1964).

Strauss, B.S., Blaufox, M.D.: Estimation of residual urine and urine flow rates without urethral catheterization. J. nucl. Med. **11**, 81–84 (1970).

Sturman, M.F., Moses, D.C., Beierwaltes, W.H., Harrison, T.S., Ice, R.D., Dorr, R.P.: Radiocholesterol adrenal images for the localization of pheochromocytoma. Surg. Gynec. Obstet. **138**, 177–180 (1974).

Summers, R.E., Concannon, J.P., Weil, C., Cole, Ch.: Determination of simultaneous effective renal plasma flow and glomerular filtration rate with ^{131}I-ortho-iodohippurate and ^{125}I-allyl inulin. J. Lab. clin. Med. **69**, 919–926 (1967).

Sy, W.M.: Bone scan in primary hyperparathyroidism. J. nucl. Med. **15**, 1089–1091 (1974).

Taplin, G.V.: Development of the use of radiopharmaceuticals in clinical nephrology. In: Progress in Nuclear Medicine, Chapter 1, Volume 2 (Blaufox, M.D., ed.), pp. 2–9. Baltimore: University Park Press 1972

Tashima, Ch.K., Lee, W.Y., Leong, A.: Tumor blood-flow study to measure response to treatment. J. nucl. Med. **15**, 463 (1974).

Tauxe, W.N.: Digital computer processing of radioisotope sciniscan matrices. J. Amer. med. Ass. **204**, 283–289 (1968).

Tauxe, W.N., Hunt, J.C.: Evaluation of renal function by isotope techniques. Med. Clin. N. Amer. **50**, 937–955 (1966).

Tauxe, W.N., Maher, F.T., Taylor, W.F.: Effective renal plasma flow: estimation from theoretical volumes of distribution of intravenously injected ^{131}I Orthoiodohippurate. Mayo Clin. Proc. **46**, 524–531 (1971).

II. Tests of Renal Function. In: Physicians Desk Reference for Radiology and Nuclear Medicine (Blaufox, M.D. and Freeman, L.M., Edit. Consultants), pp. 10–13. Oradell, New Jersey: Medical Economics Co. 1973.

Tønnesen, K.H., Munck, O., Hald, T., Mogensen, P., Wolf, H.: Influence on the Radiorenogram of variation in skin to kidney distance and the clinical importance hereof. Paper presented at the International Symposium: Radionuclides in Nephrology, Berlin, 1974.

Vernon, P., Glass, H.I.: An off-line digital system for use with a gamma camera. Phys. in Med. Biol. **16**, 405–415 (1971).

Vitye, B., LeBel, E.: Determination of renal plasma flow by a single injection of 131 I-Orthoiodohippurate and two blood samples: evaluation of the precision of this method. J. nucl. Med. **10**, 735–736 (1969).

Viville, C., Methlin, G., Grob, J.C.: La valeur de la scintigraphic quantitative au bichlorure de mercure dans l'appreciation de la fonction separee des deux reins. A propos de 55 observations. J. Urol. Néphrol. **79**, 1–16 (1972).

Vogeli, B., Riedwyl, H., Donath, A., Oetliker, O.: Comparison of glomerular filtration rate and effective renal plasma flow determinations obtained by a single injection technique and by means of a standard clearance technique in children. Acta paediat. scand. **60**, 528–532 (1971).

Wagenknecht, L.V., Knuth, O.E., Madsen, P.O.: Compensatory renal hyperfunction in the dog evaluated by continuous isotope clearance determinations. Invest. Urol. **8**, 502–506 (1971).

Wagner, H.N., Jr.: Radiomercurials in the study of renovascular hypertension. Postgrad. Med. **40**, 314–319 (1966).

Wallace, J.M., Throne, B.J.: Low-cost isotope carrier. Radiology **111**, 222 (1974).

Wang, Yen: Regional renogram: a screening test for renal hypertension evaluation. Arch. intern. Med. **134**, 463–466 (1974).

Wax, S.H.: Radioisotope uptake in experimental hydronephrosis. J. Urol. (Baltimore) **99**, 497–505 (1968).

Wax, S.H.: The abnormal radiorenogram: B. The renogram in urinary tract obstruction. In: Progress in Nuclear Medicine, Chapter 12, Volume 2 (Blaufox, M.D., ed.), pp. 259–273. Baltimore: University Park Press 1972.

Webber, M.M., Corbus, H.F.: Image communication by telephone. J. nucl. Med. **13**, 379–381 (1972).

Webber, M.M., Pollak, E.W., Victery, W., Cragin, M., Resnick, L.H., Grollman, J.H., Jr.: Thrombosis detection by radionuclide particle (MAA) entrapment: Correlation with fibrinogen uptake and venography. Radiology **3**, 645–650 (1974).

Weber, D.A., Keyes, J.W., Jr., Landman, S., Wilson, G.A.: Comparison of Tc^{99m} Polyphosphate and F^{18} for Bone Imaging. Amer. J. Roentgenol. **121**, 184–190 (1974).

Wedeen, R.P., Blaufox, M.D.: The normal renogram. In: Progress in Nuclear Medicine, Chapter 7, Volume 2 (Blaufox, M.D., ed.), pp. 107–146. Baltimore: University Park Press 1972.

Wedeen, R.P., Jernow, H.I.: Autoradiographic study of cellular transport of Hippuran-125I in the rat nephron. Amer. J. Physiol. **214**, 776–785 (1968).

Weiss, E.R., Blahd, W.H., Krishnamurthy, G.T., Winston, M.A.: The diagnosis of renal transplant rejection in association with acute tubular necrosis using the scintillation camera. J. Urol. (Baltimore) **107**, 917–921 (1972).

Weiss, E.R., Blahd, W.H., Winston, M.A., Hartenbower, D.L., Koppel, M., Thomas, P.B.: Scintillation camera in the evaluation of renal transplants. J. nucl. Med. **11**, 69–77 (1970).

Weiss, E.R., Winston, M.A., Krishnamurthy, G.T., Hartenbower, D.L., Blahd, W.H., Thomas, P.B.: Ureteral kinking and hydronephrosis in a transplanted kidney mimicking the rejection phenomenon. J. nucl. Med. **12**, 43–46 (1971).

Westerman, B.: Quantitation of the output of a scintillation camera in dynamic studies. Phys. in Med. Biol. **14**, 39–44 (1969).

Wilkiemeyer, R.M., Boyce, W.H., Malek, R.S.: Validity of the intravenous pyelogram in assessment of renal function. Surg. Gynec. Obstet. **135**, 897–900 (1972).

Wilson, D.M., Apter, J.T., Schwartz, F.D.: A model for measuring renal blood flow from plasma disappearance of iodopyracet. J. appl. Physiol. **28**, 79–88 (1970).

Winchell, H.S., Lin, M.S., Shipley, B., Sargent, T., Katchalsky-Katzir, A.: Localization of polypeptide caseidin in the renal cortex: a new radioisotope carrier for renal studies. J. nucl. Med. **12**, 678–682 (1971).

Winkel, K. zum, Harbst, H., Kishore Birendra Das, Newiger, Th.: Applications of radionuclides in renal transplantation. Semin. nucl. Med. **4**, 169–186 (1974).

Winkel, K. zum, Jost, H., Motzkus, F., Venohr, H., Golde, G.: Dynamic and morphologic examination with the scintillation camera and data processing. In: Radionuclides in Nephrology (Blaufox, M.D. and Funck-Bretano, J.-L., eds.), pp. 247–266. New York: Grune & Stratton 1972.

Winston, M.A., Halpern, S.E., Weiss, E.R., Endow, J.S., Blahd, W.H.: A critical evaluation of ^{99m}Tc-Fe-Ascorbic acid complex as a renal scanning agent. J. nucl. Med. **12**, 171–175 (1972).

Winter, Ch.C.: Renogram and other radioisotope tests in the diagnosis of renal hypertension. Amer. J. Surg. **107**, 43–49 (1964).

Winter, Ch.C., Myers, W.G.: I-125, a new radioisotope for the labeled Hippuran renogram. J. Urol. (Baltimore) **88**, 100–102 (1962).

Wisenbaugh, P.E., Clark, R.E., Wills, N.E., Jelliffe, R.W.: The radioisotope renogram in dogs with experimental renal artery stenosis. Amer. Heart J. **69**, 655–667 (1965).

Woodruff, M.W., Kibler, R.S., Bender, M.A., Blau, M.: HG-203 Neohydrin kidney photoscan: an adjuvant to diagnosis of renal disease. J. Urol. (Baltimore) **89**, 746–751 (1963).

Yeh, Shin-Hwa, Kriss, J.P.: Distribution and scintiphotography of a new complex, pentavalent Technetium-99m citrate: studies in the rodent. J. nucl. Med. **8**, 666–677 (1967).

Urological Ultrasonography

G.R. LEOPOLD and L.B. TALNER

With 22 Figures

A. Introduction

Imaging of urinary tract structures by reflected ultrasonic pulses has been in use for less than a decade. Only within the past 5 years or so has the technique developed to the point where it can be considered an important and useful examination in patients with some types of urinary tract disease. The method adapts well to the examination of the kidneys and bladder since satisfactory studies can be obtained in nearly all patients, regardless of age or body build. It is painless and in light of current knowledge, without harm to the patient. Although used extensively in gynecologic conditions and in all phases of pregnancy for nearly 20 years, no case of physical or genetic damage from ultrasound has yet been reported. Experimental studies have similarly failed to demonstrate chromosomal aberrations or other signs of genetic damage, even from prolonged exposure to the power levels utilized in diagnostic instruments (BOBROW, 1971).

Ultrasonic images (often called echograms) display tissue differences not possible with conventional roentgenograms. For example, a renal cyst, a dilated renal pelvis, and the urinary bladder can be clearly distinguished from adjacent structures. This unique capability of differentiating fluid-containing from solid tissues makes ultrasound particularly well suited to the evaluation of renal mass lesions.

However rewarding this method of examination has become, the future holds even more promise. Recent refinements in image recording have permitted much more subtle interface detection, resulting in remarkable improvement in resolution. It is now frequently possible to visualize the kidneys and urinary bladder of the fetus during the last months of gestation. With the increasing desire to examine the fetus in utero, ultrasound will assume an expanding role. There is little doubt that technological improvements will continue to widen the scope and applications of ultrasound in urologic diagnosis.

B. Basic Principles

I. Physics

The central element of any ultrasonic instrument is its transducer which functions both as a sender of pulses and a receiver of reflected pulses (echoes) from tissue interfaces. Most transducers are composed of a synthetic, polarized, ceramic, crystalline material such as lead zirconate titanate or barium titanate. These materials are piezoelectric; that is, when an electrical voltage is impressed across it, the crystal alters structure slightly, causing energy to be emitted in the form of high frequency sound waves. For medical diagnostic applications, the desired frequency is in the range of 1–10 million cps (1–10 megaHz) with 2.25 megaHz representing a commonly available frequency on commercial instruments. The transducer is stimulated between 500–1000 times/s by an alternating current, and the resultant pulses are approximately 1 μs in duration. Consequently, the transducer spends the great bulk of its time receiving echoes from within the tissue being examined. In general, echoes are generated from tissue interfaces when a change occurs in physical density. Homogeneous structures, be they cystic or solid, will return relatively few echoes while the edges of organs and masses or those with complex internal structure will produce many reflections. The term "sonolucent" refers to the easy passage of ultrasonic waves through a structure or organ. By determining the time elapsed from transmission of a pulse to the reception of an echo, the distance from the transducer to the interface in question may be accurately measured—provided the velocity of sound in the medium is known and remains constant.

Upon reaching the transducer, the returning echo strikes and deforms the crystal, thereby generating a small electric pulse proportional to the strength of the returning echo. The pulses are displayed on a cathode ray oscilloscope which usually has a scale permitting a direct reading of distance from the transducer to the reflecting interface.

II. A-Mode Display

There are two forms of data display in common use for urological ultrasonography. The simplest is the A-mode display, in which echoes are shown as vertical spikes of varying amplitude along a horizontal time base. This is a one dimensional representation of the acoustic interfaces along the line of sight of the transducer. As such, it is useful only when the tissue or organ being examined has been localized precisely within the body. For example, A-mode alone can reveal considerable diagnostic information about a mass previously localized by palpation or x-ray studies. The instruments needed for A-mode examination are much less expensive than those used for the B-scans to be described below.

III. B-Mode and Gray Scale

In most cases it is desirable to obtain a two-dimensional image of the underlying anatomy. This format, known as a "B-scan," is achieved by reducing the echoes to bright dots (rather than spikes). The transducer, mounted on a rigid mechanical arm, is manually guided along a preselected path on the surface of the patient. The signals received are displayed on the oscilloscope in correct spatial relationship to one another by means of a system of potentiometers. In order to retain information from various transducer positions during the scanning maneuvers, most conventional instruments employ an oscilloscope coated with a persistence phosphor. The image gradually builds up on the screen as progressively more sightings are received. Upon completion of each scan, which ordinarily takes from 20–30 s, the oscilloscope is photographed for a permanent record. Recently, a more sophisticated recording apparatus has been introduced, replacing the phosphor coated oscilloscopic screen with a television scan converter. This innovation allows the recording of previously rejected low intensity echoes (such as those emanating from the renal parenchyma), and the final display is taken from a television screen. As many as eight or nine separate intensity levels of echoes may be distinguished, resulting in considerable enhancement of tissue discrimination. These scans are usually termed "gray scale" studies and are so designated in the legends of this chapter. Gray scale scanning is highly preferable to conventional imaging.

Under ordinary circumstances a parallel series of scans is obtained spaced at 1–2 cm intervals over the area of interest. A second series oriented at a right angle to the first is often helpful in conceiving the anatomy in three dimensions.

C. Method of Examination

When the kidneys or upper retroperitoneal space are being examined, the patient is ordinarily placed in the prone position. The kidneys are close to the surface and interfering effects of bowel gas are eliminated. The study begins with a series of transverse scans starting at the level of the iliac crest and proceeds cephalad at 1–2 cm intervals until the lungs preclude further visualization. In order to successfully pass sound into the body, a coupling agent such as mineral oil is applied to the skin of the back. During the performance of the scan the technologist rocks the transducer back and forth in the scan plane, thereby achieving perpendicularity to a maximum number of interfaces within the tissue being examined.

Following completion of the transverse scans, the instrument is reoriented to record a series of sagittal scans over each flank. Although such scans are generally made parallel to the midplane, oblique scans are sometimes used to reproduce the axis of the kidney and thereby estimate its length more accurately.

When the urinary bladder is to be examined the patient is studied supine. Prone scans are of little value because of the shielding effect of the bony pelvis. Visualization of the prostate and bladder base is enhanced by conducting the study with a distended urinary bladder. As with most B-scan procedures, two series of scans oriented 90° to each other are necessary to adequately survey the area of interest.

Under ordinary circumstances the examination of either the kidneys or bladder takes no longer than 20 min. For obvious practical reasons, the examination is greatly facilitated by first reviewing a recent intravenous urogram. Abnormalities discovered on the ultrasonic scans should be directly compared with the radiographs to insure that the proper regions have been examined in detail. By so doing, the maximum diagnostic benefit from both studies is achieved.

D. Normal Anatomy

I. Kidney-Transverse Anatomy

At present ultrasound is the only widely used technique offering a display of renal anatomy in transverse section. Computerized axial tomography, still evolving, also shows transverse anatomy. Transverse

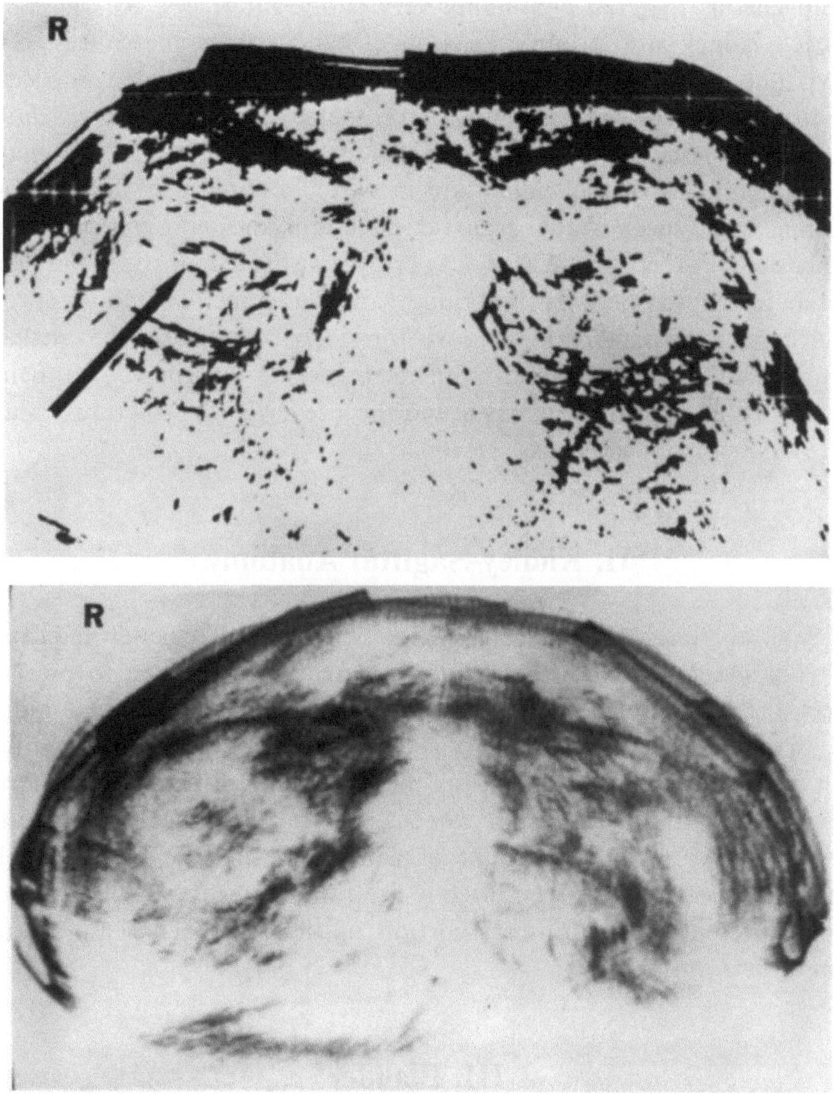

A

B

Fig. 1. (A) Prone, transverse scan. Normal kidneys. *R* indicates right side of patient on this and all subsequent transverse scans. *Arrow* indicates caliceal echoes within sonolucent renal parenchyma of right kidney. (B) Prone, transverse scan (gray scale). Normal right kidney. Previous left nephrectomy. Parenchymal as well as caliceal echoes now apparent

scans of the kidneys reveal them to be round or oval in external contour (Figs. 1A, 1B). The bulk of renal parenchyma, using conventional equipment and average sensitivity settings, appears free of echoes. This appearance is also typical of organs such as the liver and spleen, and indicates only that the parenchyma of these organs is composed of relatively homogeneous material containing very subtle interfaces. At the center of each kidney is a strong collection of echoes from the calices, renal pelvis, and major vessels entering the renal hilus. An accurate comparison of renal size is seldom possible from transverse scans since grossly different portions of each kidney often lie on the same transverse plane. The upper poles of the kidney are in close proximity to the vertebral column, while more caudal transverse sections show progressive lateral displacement of varying degree. Lower pole scans demonstrate the psoas muscle interposed between the kidney and the spine. The vertebral column casts a characteristic shadow anteriorly, caused by the virtually complete reflection of sound from its posterior margin. Consequently the aorta, the inferior vena cava, and the prevertebral structures cannot be evaluated from the back.

II. Kidney-Sagittal Anatomy

Sagittal (longitudinal) scans of the kidney give a better indication of renal size but, as noted previously, care must be taken to precisely select the true long axis of the organ (Figs. 2A, 2B). Actual kidney length can then be measured very accurately and without the magnification distortion which renders x-ray measurements difficult. The internal caliceal pattern is easily appreciated as in transverse scans. Above the right kidney a variable amount of sonolucent liver is usually visible while the spleen may be seen directly atop the left kidney. Unless distension is present, the extrarenal portion of the renal pelvis and ureters cannot be identified.

III. Bladder

The urine-filled bladder, examined sagittally in the supine position is shown in Fig. 3. Characteristically, its superior aspect tapers to a point which is directed toward the umbilicus. The anterior aspect of the urinary bladder is often marked by a band of artifactual echoes caused by reverberation at the strong bladder wall-urine interface. The identification of pathologic processes in the most anterior 3 cm of the bladder is often difficult because of these reverberation echoes.

The normal prostate is incompletely visualized from this suprapubic approach. In the female patient, the uterus is usually completely demon-

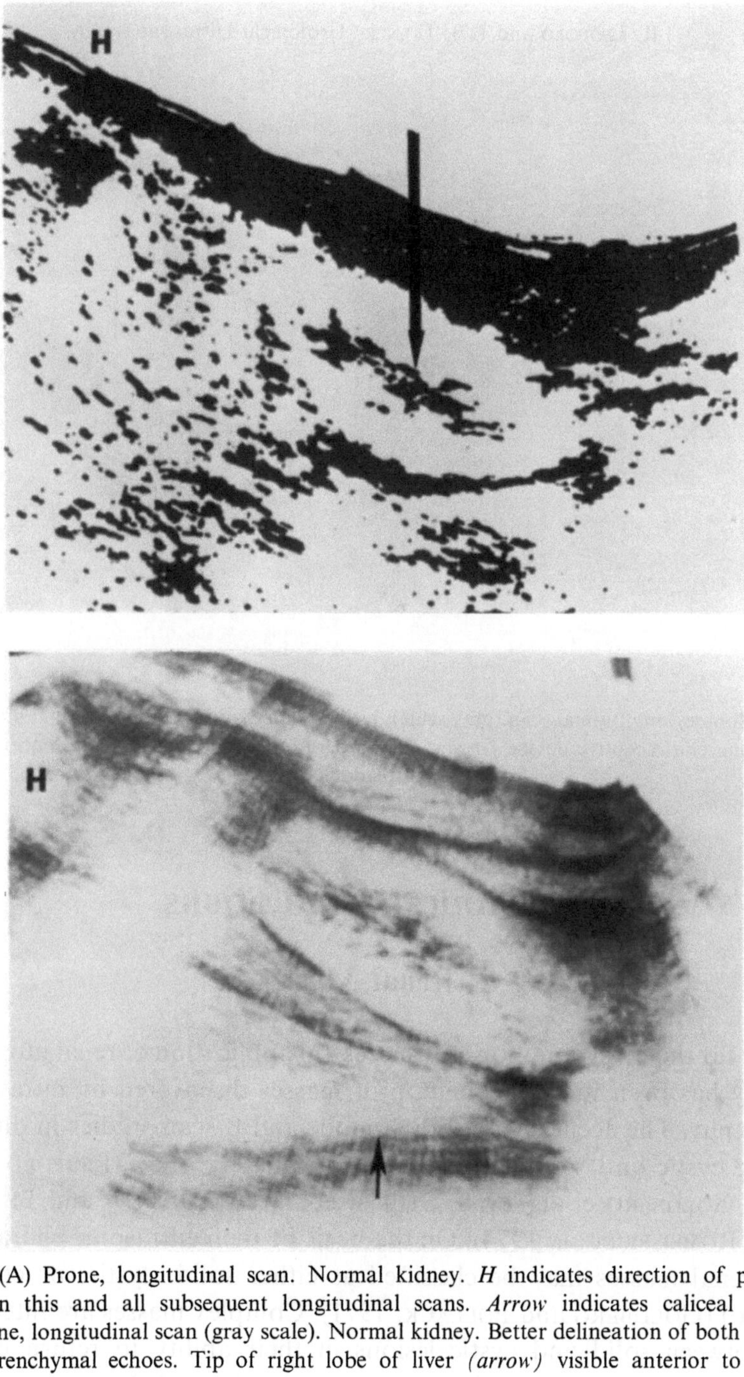

A

B

Fig. 2. (A) Prone, longitudinal scan. Normal kidney. *H* indicates direction of patient's head on this and all subsequent longitudinal scans. *Arrow* indicates caliceal echoes. (B) Prone, longitudinal scan (gray scale). Normal kidney. Better delineation of both caliceal and parenchymal echoes. Tip of right lobe of liver *(arrow)* visible anterior to kidney

strated immediately posterior to the distended urinary bladder. For this reason, ultrasonic examination of the uterus and other pelvic masses is ordinarily intentionally conducted with the bladder filled.

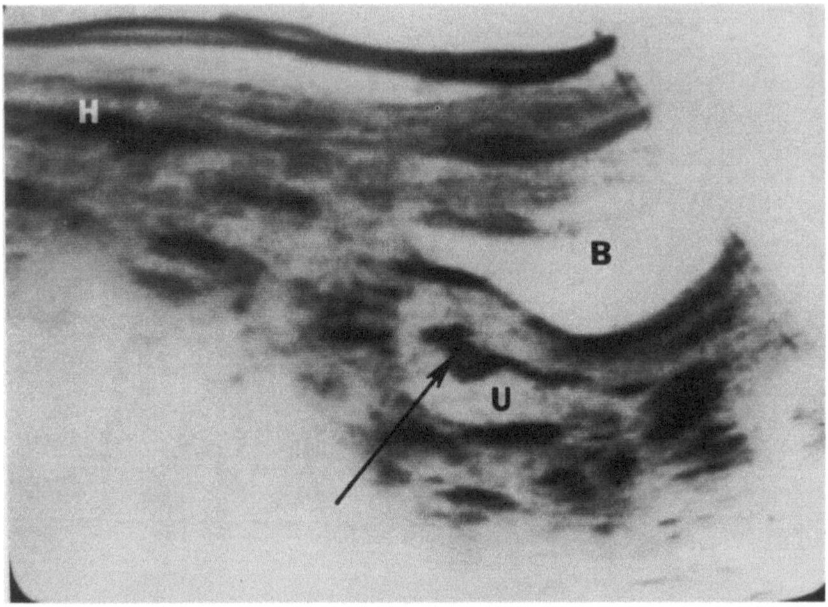

Fig. 3. Supine, longitudinal scan (gray scale). Urine filled bladder (*B*) and normal uterus (*U*) containing contraceptive device *(arrow)*. Reverberation echoes present in anterior aspect of bladder

E. Clinical Applications

I. Renal Masses

By far the most common and successful application of renal ultrasonography has been in the evaluation of masses discovered by intravenous urography. The accuracy of both A-mode and B-scan studies in differentiating cystic and solid lesions is approximately 95% (LEOPOLD et al., 1973; GOLDBERG et al., 1968; STUBER et al., 1972; SMITH and BENNETT, 1975; ROMEISER et al., 1974). On the basis of their ultrasonic characteristics, renal masses may be classified as either solid, cystic, or complex (mixed) (GOLDBERG and POLLACK, 1971). Complex masses are intermediate between solid and cystic lesions in their ability to return echoes.

If A-mode alone is being used, the location of the mass must be established before the scanning procedure, either by palpation, fluoroscopy, radionuclide imaging, previous B-scan study, or, as in most instances, urography. The transducer is aimed in the predetermined direction and the depth of the mass from the skin as well as its internal

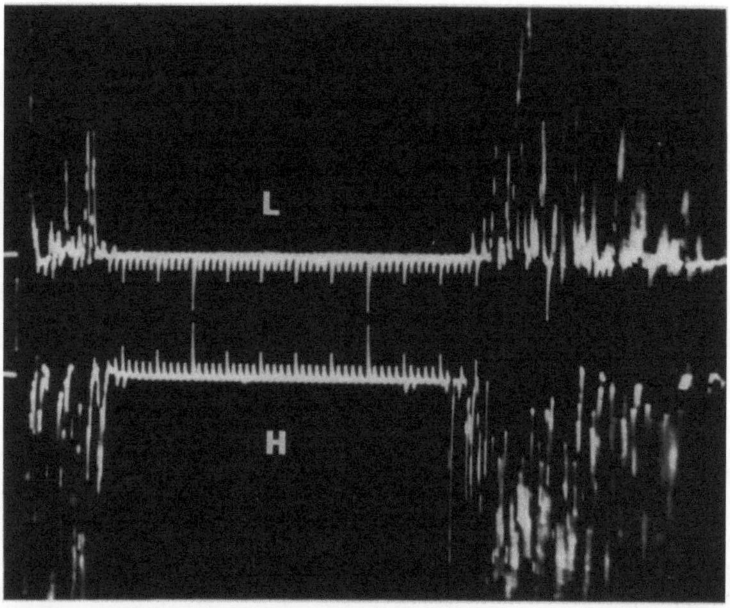

A

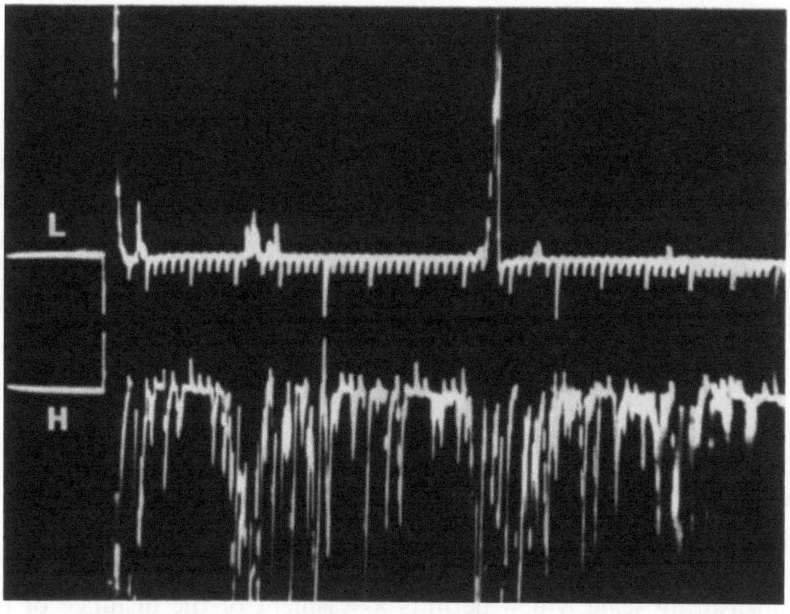

B

Fig. 4. (A) A-mode examination of renal cyst. Strong echoes mark near and far surfaces of cyst, with no intervening echoes at low gain (*L*). At higher gain (*H*) cyst remains echo-free. (B) A-mode examination of solid renal carcinoma. Although low gain study (*L*) shows few internal echoes, far wall echo is much diminished. High gain study (*H*) brings out multiple internal echoes, indicating solid nature of mass

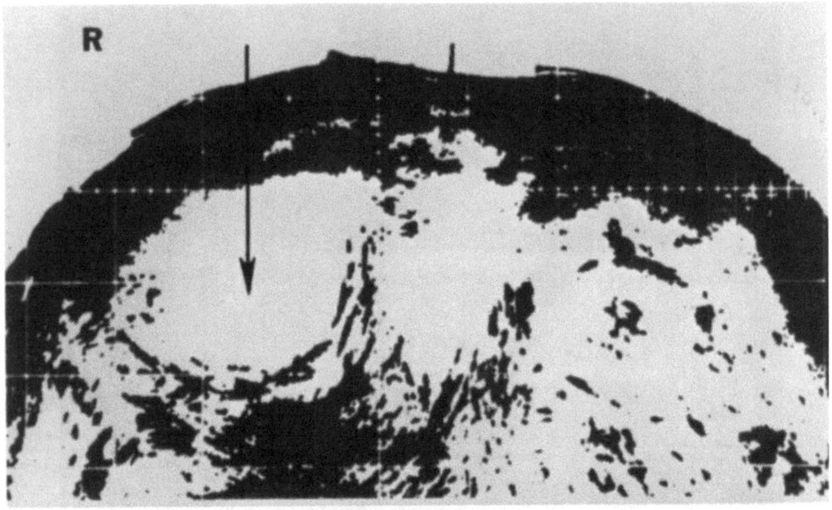

A

Fig. 5. (A) Prone, transverse scan. *Arrow* points to center of 8 cm right renal cyst. Normal left kidney also shown. (B) Nephrotomogram demonstrates characteristic findings of renal cyst, right upper pole. (C) Following percutaneous puncture, injected contrast material outlines smooth cyst wall

ultrasonic characteristics are noted. Photography of the A-mode tracing is ordinarily performed to provide a permanent record.

Most workers prefer B-scan analysis (often combined with A-mode examination) because of the increased anatomical information obtained (KING, 1972; SCHRECK and HOLMES, 1970; MOUNTFORD et al., 1971; DOUST et al., 1973). Not only can the size and location of the mass within the kidney be ascertained, but its relationship to surrounding structures such as the liver and spleen can be determined as well. This may be an important factor if percutaneous aspiration is anticipated.

1. Cysts

An A-mode tracing of a typical renal cyst is shown in Fig. 4A. The top portion of the tracing is obtained at normal instrument settings and shows the anterior and posterior margins of the cyst superimposed on a measuring scale which permits assessment of the distance of these interfaces from the skin surface. The interior of the cyst, because it contains no reflecting interfaces, appears empty. On the bottom trace another examination has been made in exactly the same position with an increased sensitivity (high gain) setting that allows detection of very subtle echoes. Even at this enhanced sensitivity level, the center of the

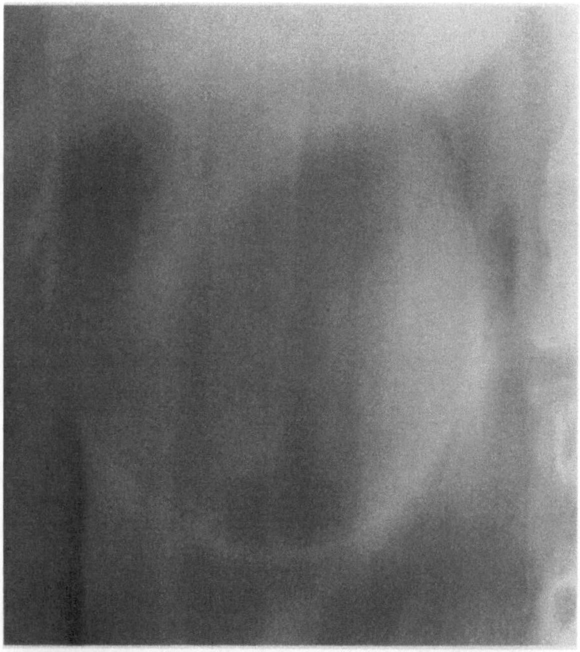

B

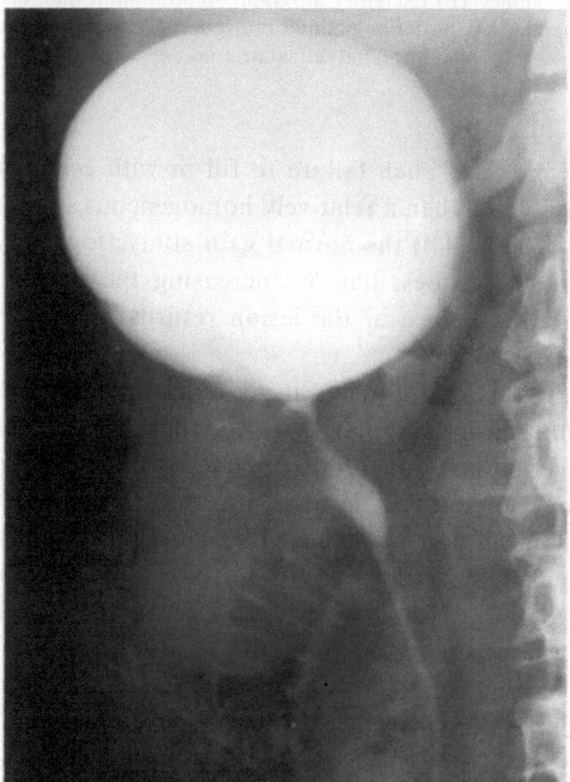

Fig. 5B and C C

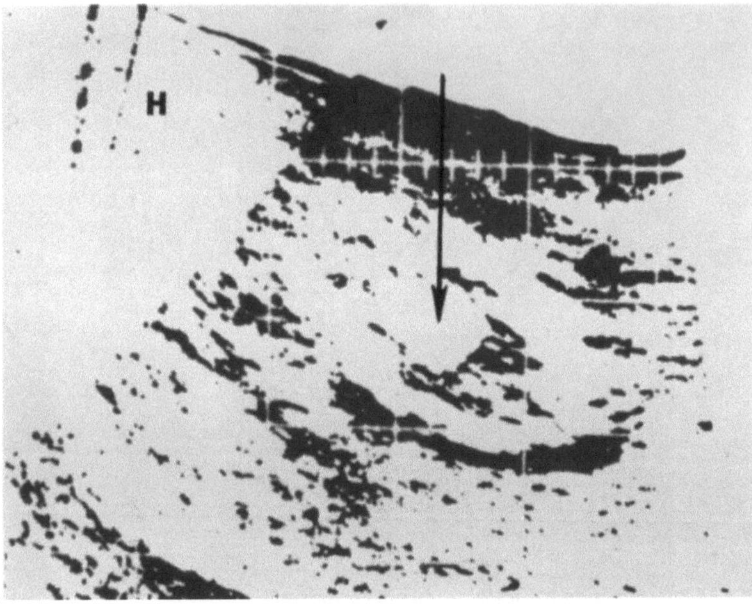

A

Fig. 6. (A) Prone, longitudinal scan. 3 cm peripelvic cyst *(arrow)* distorts central caliceal echo pattern of left kidney. (B) Excretory urogram. Smooth impression on left renal pelvis. (C) Renal arteriogram, left posterior oblique projection. Peripelvic cyst causes spreading of ventral and dorsal arteries *(arrows)*

cyst remains echo free. Such failure to fill in with echoes allows cystic-solid differentiation. When a relatively homogeneous solid mass is examined by A-mode (Fig. 4B) the normal gain study (top) may also appear remarkably free of echoes, but on increasing the sensitivity level, the complex internal structure of the lesion returns multiple small echoes, indicating its true nature.

Utilizing the B-scan approach, it is ordinarily possible to completely outline the contour of a renal cyst, whether it is peripheral (Fig. 5) or peripelvic (Fig. 6). As mentioned previously, correlation with the intravenous urogram is advisable to ensure that the two methods are describing the same lesion. Just as with A-mode examination, high as well as low sensitivity settings are useful in establishing the consistency of renal masses. In B-mode display, cysts are characterized by an absence of internal echoes, sharp margination, and increased transmission through and beyond the lesion. The latter is manifested by an excessive amount of echoes piling up on the far side of the lesion. When a mass satisfies these three criteria its chances of being a renal cyst are 95%. With present day equipment the lower limit of resolution for a cyst is believed

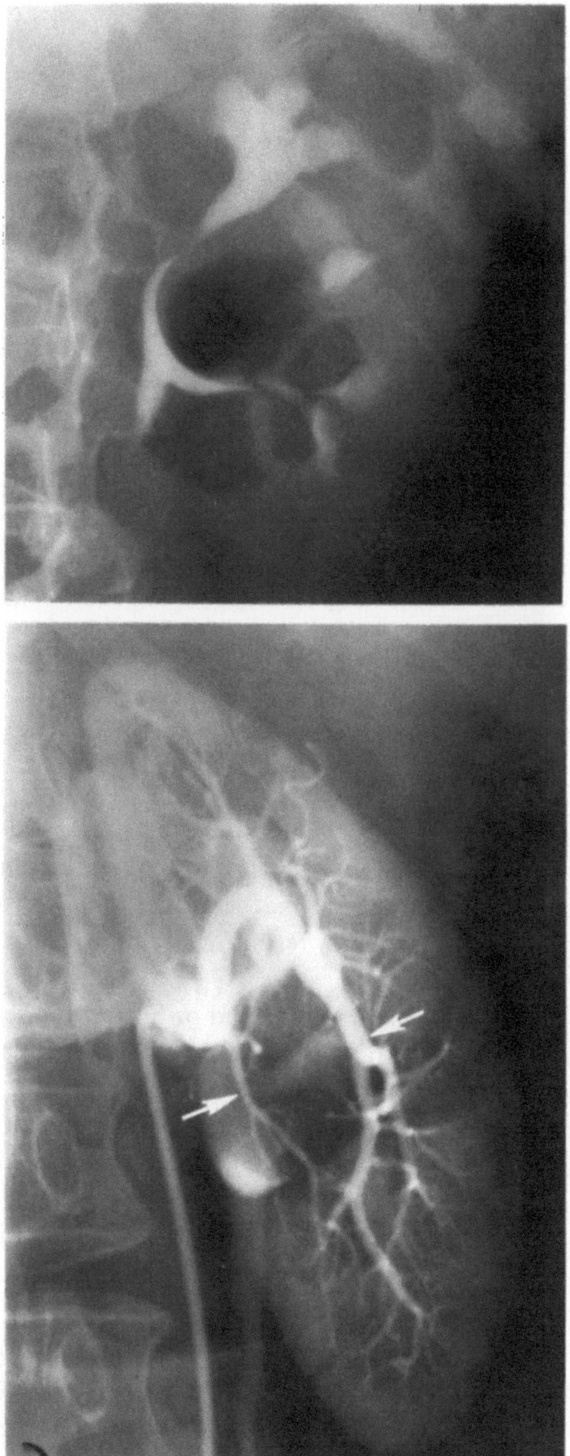

B

Fig. 6B and C C

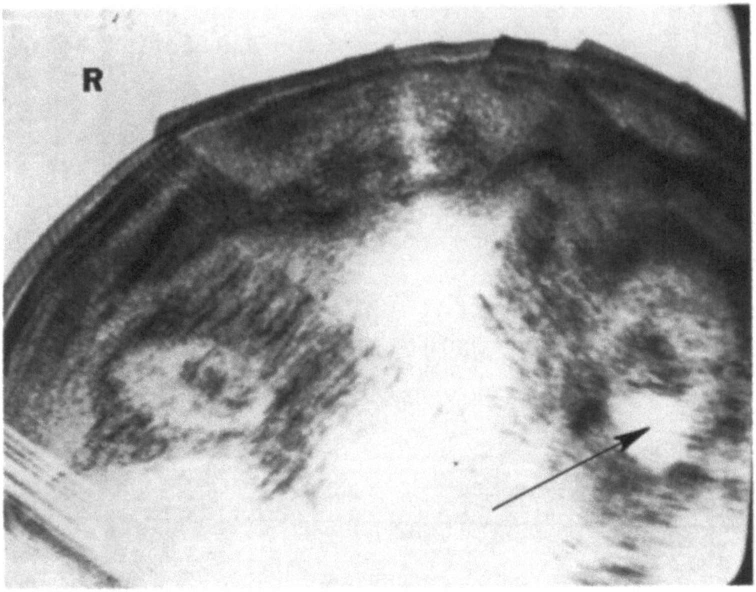

Fig. 7. Prone, transverse scan (gray scale). 2-cm cyst *(arrow)* arising from anterior surface, left kidney. Because of small size, lesion could easily be overlooked on intravenous urography. Lower pole of normal right kidney also shown

to be a diameter of 2 cm (Fig. 7). Because the lungs and rib cage are variably superimposed on the upper poles, lower pole lesions are slightly easier to demonstrate than those in the upper pole. Visualization of small lesions will be enhanced if respiration can be suspended during the scan.

Polycystic kidneys are easily recognized on ultrasonic scans (HOLMES, 1971) (Fig. 8). The kidneys are usually enlarged, irregular in outline, and contain many cysts of varying size. Since the method is solely dependent on anatomy rather than function, a specific diagnosis can almost always be made, even when the patient has overt renal failure. When polycystic disease is uncovered, complete scanning of the liver should be performed because of the associated hepatic cysts in 25% of patients. Cysts of the spleen and pancreas may also be demonstrated on occasion. Some have advocated ultrasonic scanning of the families of such patients to detect preclinical states (HOLMES, 1971). At its present level of development, however, ultrasound scanning is not as sensitive as high-dose nephrotomography or angiography in the diagnosis of *early* polycystic kidney disease.

2. Percutaneous Cyst Puncture

It is often practical to combine the ultrasonic study with percutaneous cyst aspiration to obtain fluid for cytological and chemical analysis (ASHER and LEOPOLD, 1972; LEOPOLD et al., 1973). Percutaneous aspiration may be done in conjunction with either fluoroscopic or ultrasonic localization, or both (DOUST and MAKLAD, 1973). The combination of clear fluid, negative cytologic examination, absent stainable lipid, and a smooth inner wall makes the diagnosis of renal cyst a virtual certainty (greater than 99%) (LANG, 1966, 1971a, b, 1973; KRISTENSEN et al., 1972; VON SCHREEB et al., 1967; THORNBURY, 1972; SHERWOOD and STEVENSON, 1971; LINDBLOM, 1952; LALLI, 1967; JEANS et al., 1972; STEG et al., 1971; OLSSON, 1973).

A unique ultrasonic localization method has been developed utilizing a special A-mode transducer with a hollow central core large enough to accommodate an aspiration needle (GOLDBERG and POLLACK, 1973a, b). Having localized the lesion by B-scan or some other method, the overlying skin is cleansed and local anesthetic injected. The sterile transducer is placed on the skin mark and angled until the characteristic pattern of the cyst is seen in A-mode display on the oscilloscope. The needle is advanced until its tip reaches the center of the cyst as determined from the oscilloscopic tracing. A distinct "pop" is usually felt on entering the cyst. If a steel needle is used, the tip of the needle is visualized as a strong echo within the cyst, thus facilitating placement close to its center. Some prefer to use a teflon sheath, in which case the needle tip will not be visible by ultrasound (LEOPOLD, 1973). Following aspiration of a small amount of cyst fluid for analysis, radiographic contrast material is introduced and films exposed to detect filling defects within or along the lining of the cyst. The entire procedure ordinarily takes no more than 30 min and can be performed easily on outpatients. The major advantage of the intravenous urography-ultrasound-puncture sequence is that it obviates the renal arteriogram in the vast majority of renal cysts and does not sacrifice diagnostic accuracy. Patient hospitalization, physician time, and hospital costs are minimized as well.

Although peripelvic cysts are clearly demonstrable by these techniques, some would defer percutaneous puncture because of the proximity to the major renal vessels (Fig. 6). Furthermore, such cysts are frequently multi-loculated and puncture with subsequent contrast injection may be considerably harder to interpret if only a single locule has been entered (LALLI, 1967). Care must also be taken to assure that the suspected

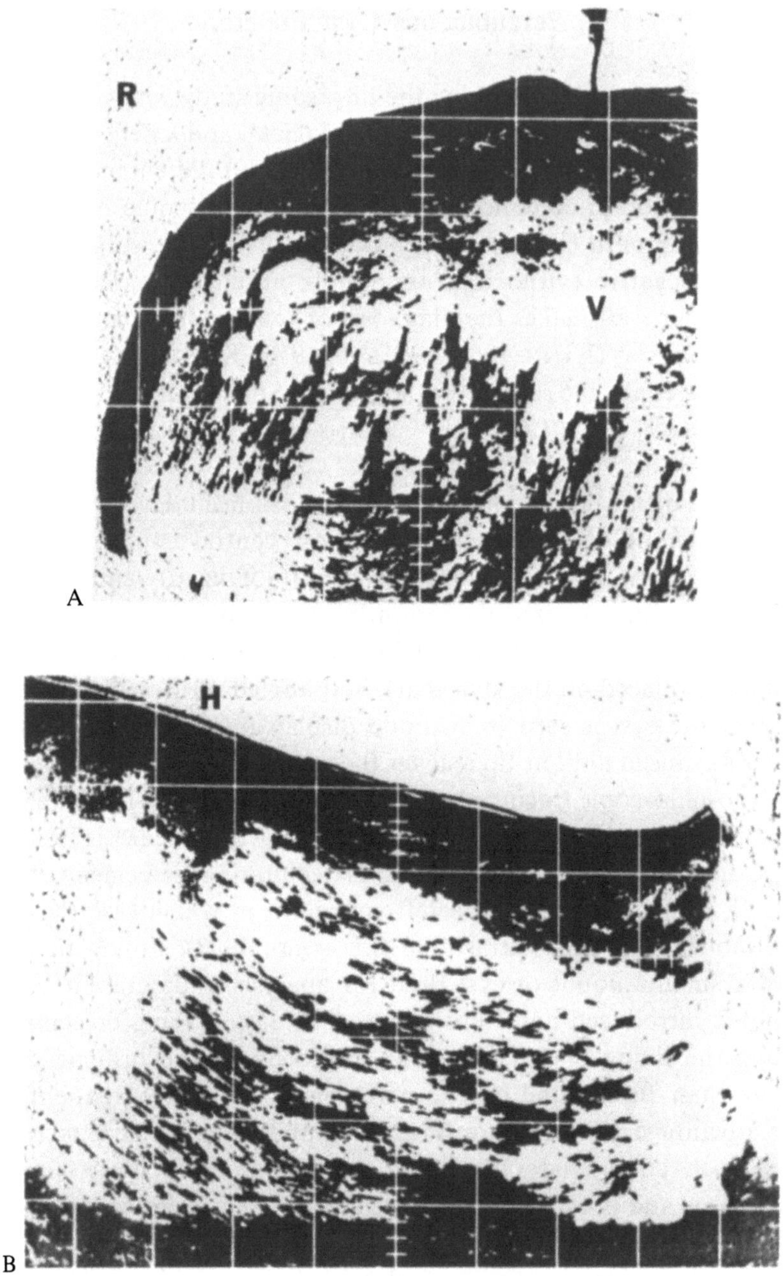

Fig. 8. (A) Prone, transverse scan. Polycystic kidneys. Normal caliceal pattern of right kidney replaced by numerous arcuate echoes produced by many cysts of varying size. V = vertebral column. (B) Prone, longitudinal scan. Polycystic right kidney greatly enlarged (18 cm long) with echo pattern as in A. (C) Late phase selective arteriogram. Typical "Swiss-cheese" pattern of polycystic renal disease

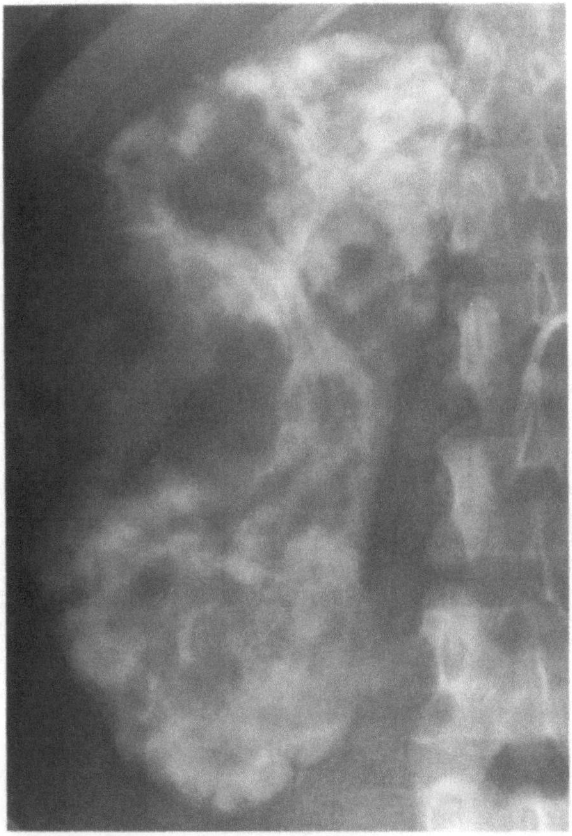

Fig. 8C

"cyst" is not a dilated renal pelvis secondary to ureteral obstruction, or a large renal artery aneurysm.

3. Complex or Solid Masses

When a renal mass shows internal echo formation or irregular margins, it is almost always something other than a cyst. Tumors commonly show a great many diffuse echoes of rather weak nature. The degree of tumor vascularity shown by angiography correlates poorly with the amount of echoes produced. Two renal tumors, one highly vascular and the other with only sparse vascularity, show similar echographic features (Figs. 9, 10). Since it may be difficult to differentiate a hypovascular carcinoma from a simple cyst angiographically, ultrasonic study is extremely helpful when such a lesion is present (McLaughlin et al., 1974).

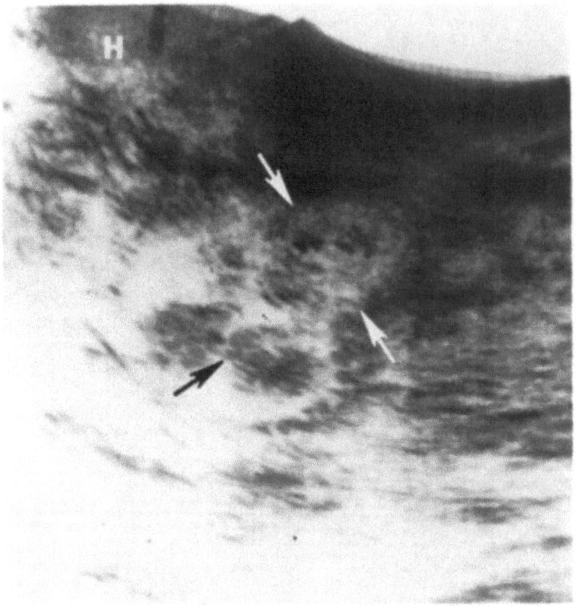

A

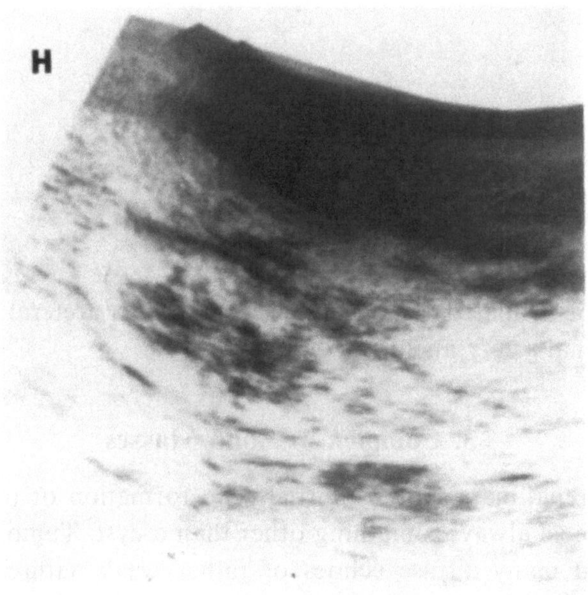

B

Fig. 9. (A) Prone, longitudinal scan (gray scale). Right renal carcinoma. Lobulated, solid mass *(white arrows)* protrudes from posterior surface of kidney. Unusually prominent caliceal echoes *(black arrow)* probably related to renal sinus lipomatosis. (B) Prone, longitudinal (gray scale). Patient's left kidney also shows accentuated central echo pattern from sinus fat accumulation. (C) Excretory urogram. Renal tumor distorts lower pole calices. Sinus lipomatosis stretches middle and upper infundibula. (D) Right renal arteriogram, left posterior oblique projection. Extremely vascular lower pole tumor extends postero-laterally into perirenal tissues

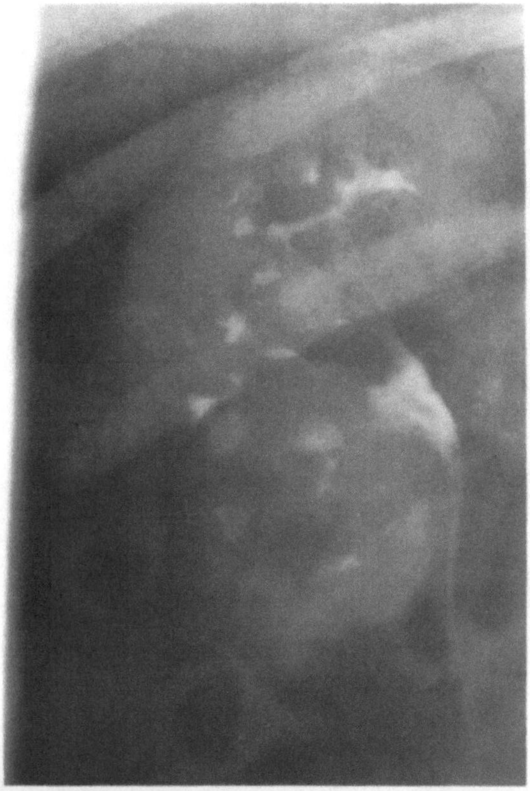

C

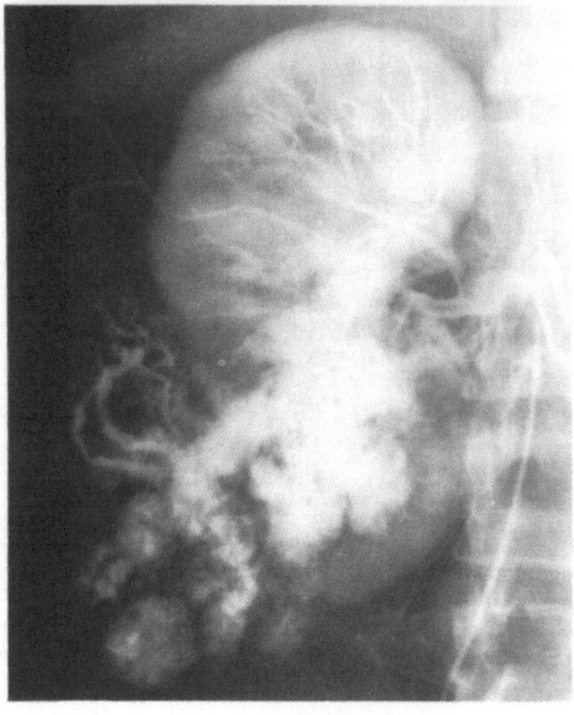

Fig. 9C and D D

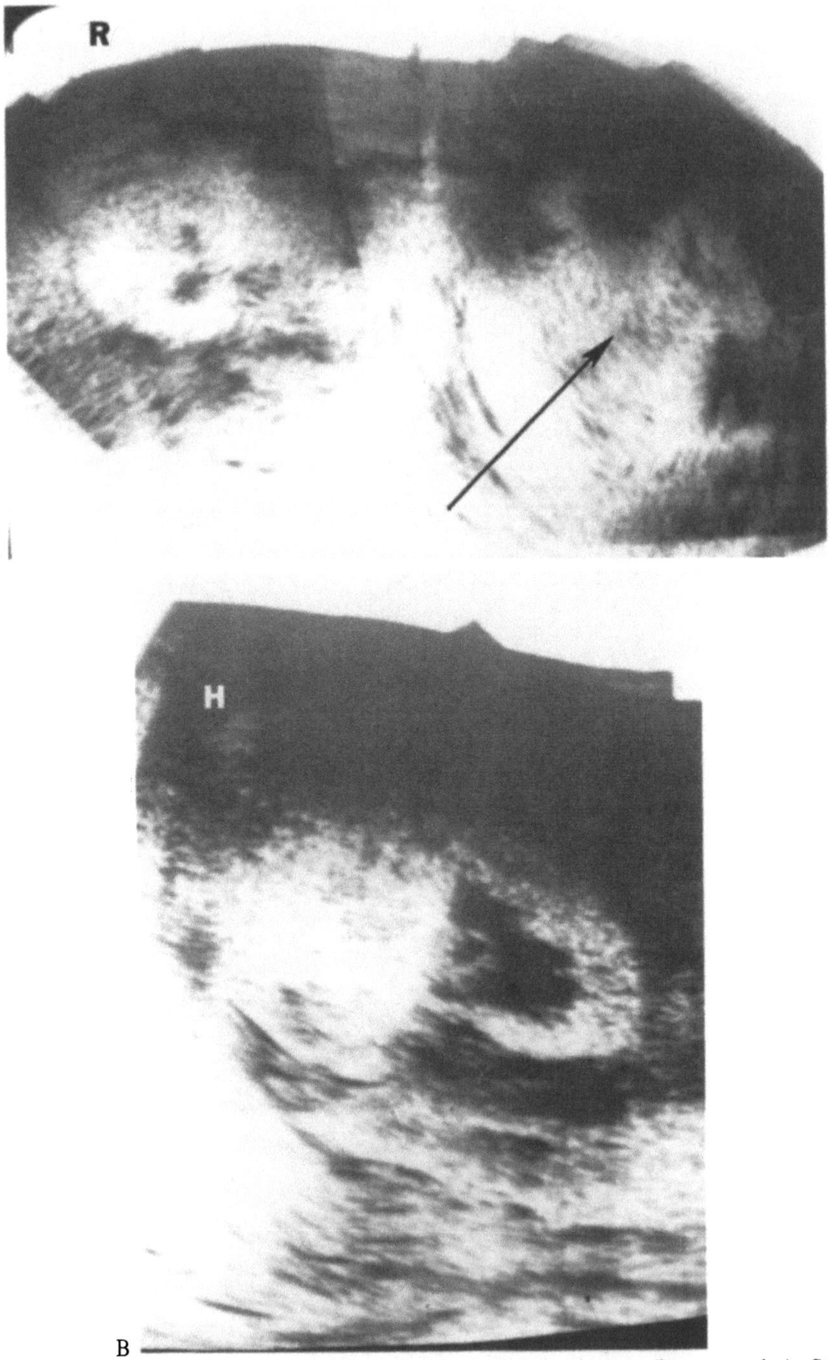

A

B

Fig. 10. (A) Prone, transverse scan (gray scale). Renal carcinoma (hypovascular). Study at level of upper pole of left kidney shows large mass *(arrow to center of mass)* containing many internal echoes. Compare with normal right kidney at same level. (B) Prone, longitudinal scan (gray scale). Entire left upper pole replaced by tumor which extends anteriorly.

C

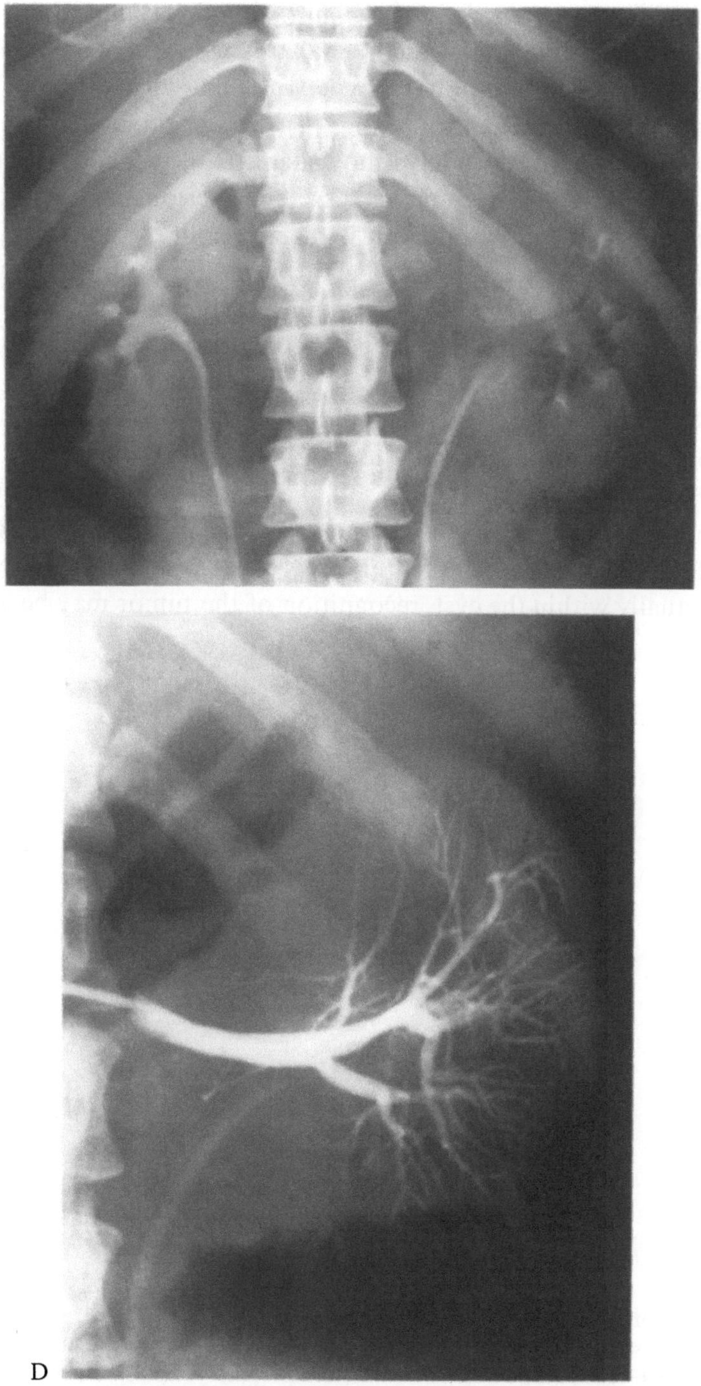

D

Fig. 10. (C) Excretory urogram. Left upper pole mass distorts calices and renal axis. (D) Left renal arteriogram. Marked hypovascularity of lesion resembles renal cyst. Echo study in this case allows distinction between solid and cystic mass

In the case of a noncystic mass, ultrasound has not been helpful thus far in differential diagnosis. Renal abscess (Fig. 11), hematoma, hemorrhagic cyst, pseudotumor (hypertrophied cortical tissue), xanthogranulomatous pyelonephritis (Fig. 12), benign tumors (Fig. 13), and renal carcinoma (Figs. 9, 10) have shown similar ultrasonic patterns. Angiography should be carried out in these solid lesions to obtain further diagnostic information. Although it is theoretically possible for a tumor to be so necrotic that it appears to be a cyst on ultrasound examination, the walls of such a lesion will be irregular and the debris within usually generates a few echoes. Should an erroneous diagnosis of cyst be made on the basis of ultrasound, puncture of the lesion will lead to the correct diagnosis.

A potentially confusing situation exists when a tumor and a cyst are present within the same kidney. If the lesions are both of sufficient size to be demonstrated by ultrasound, diagnosis will not be difficult (KING, 1972). If, however, the tumor is relatively small and located near or actually within the cyst, recognition of the tumor may be difficult.

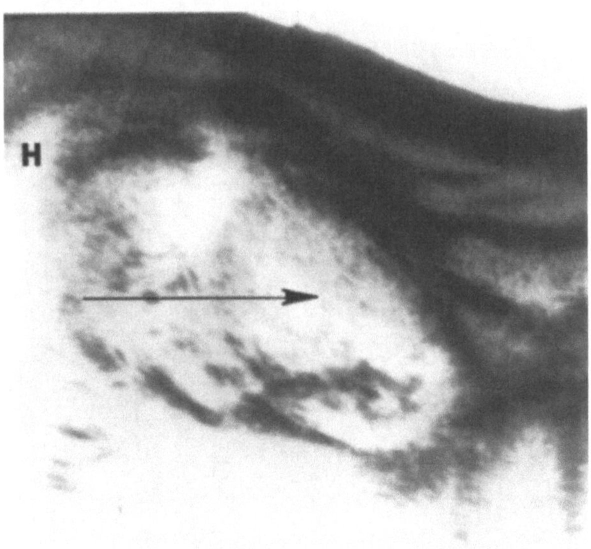

A

Fig. 11. (A) Prone, longitudinal scan (gray scale). Renal abscess in a heroin addict. Large mass *(arrow)* displaces calices anteriorly. Multiple internal echoes are present. (B) Excretory urogram. Right calices manifest minimal distortion only. Lateral kidney margin intact since abscess located posteriorly. (C) Right renal arteriogram, left posterior oblique projection. Major abnormality is stretching of arteries in central portion of kidney. No neovascularity. Diminished parenchymal opacification in region of abscess

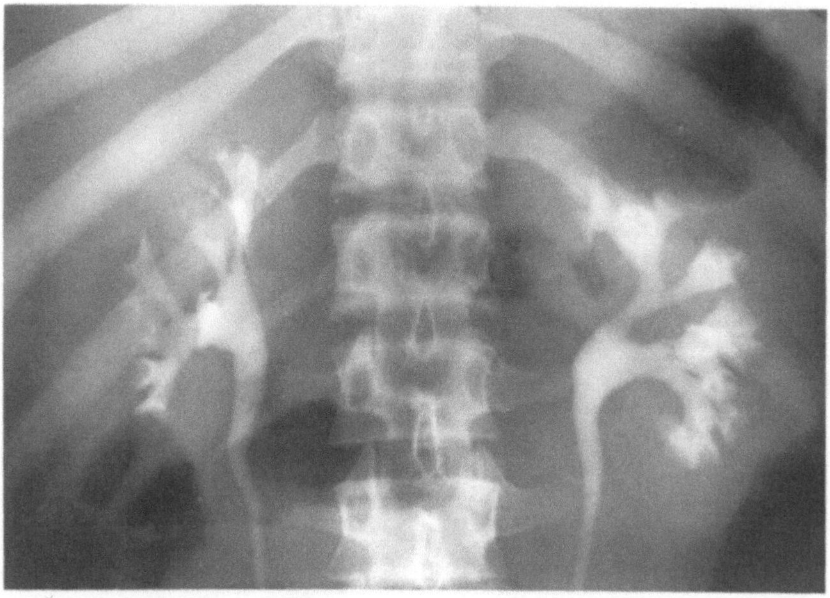

B

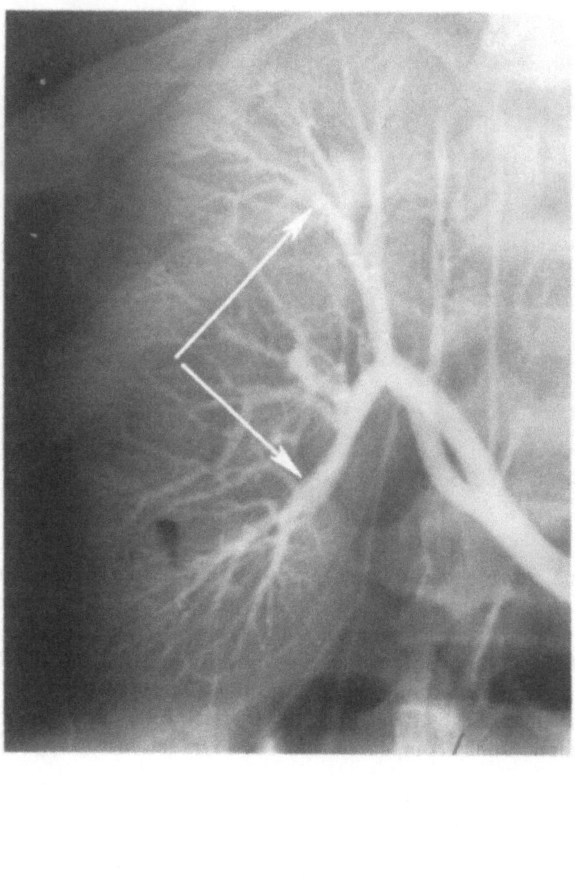

Fig. 11 B and C C

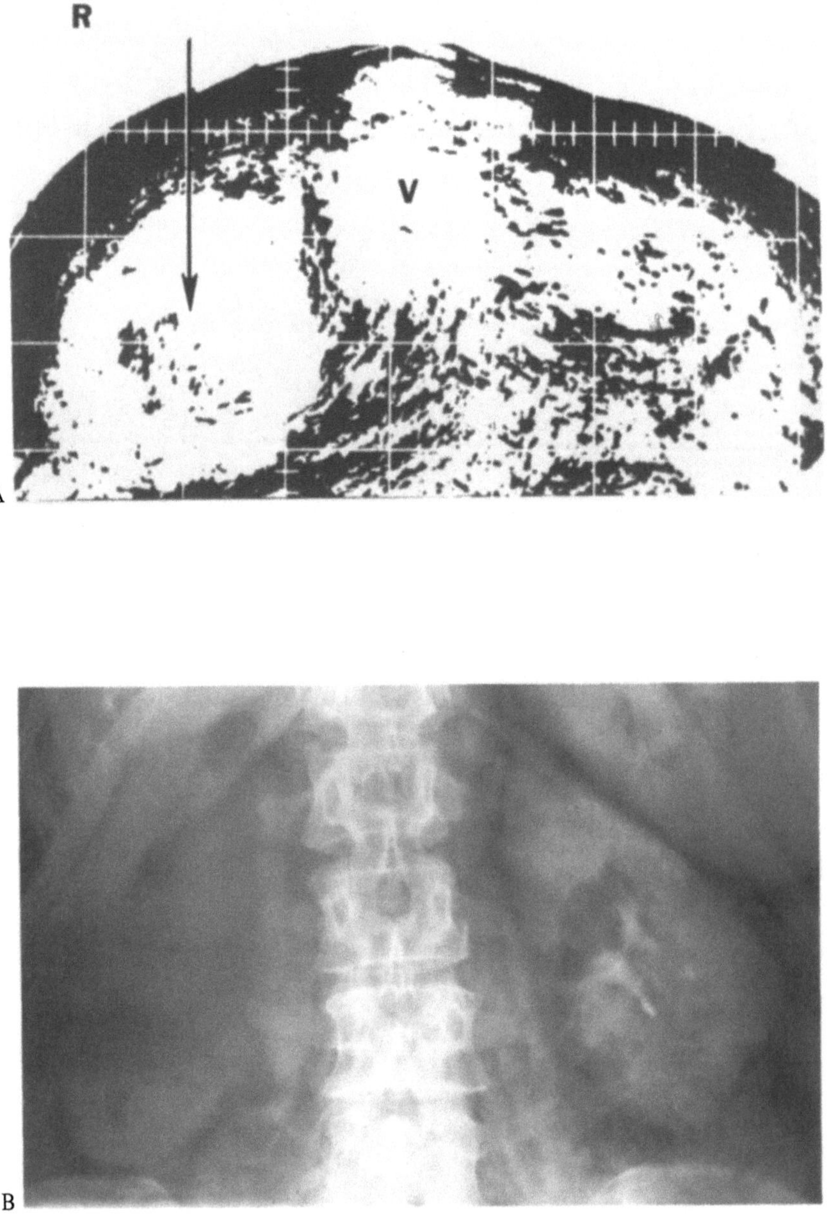

A

B

Fig. 12. (A) Prone, transverse scan. Pyonephrosis with xanthogranulomatous pyelonephritis. Right kidney *(arrow)* is enlarged and contains scattered, internal echoes. *V* = vertebral column. Differentiation from carcinoma is not possible. (B) Excretory urogram. Total nonvisualization of right kidney. Soft tissue mass in right renal fossa. No stones. (C) Right renal arteriogram, right posterior oblique projection. Upper of two renal arteries injected. Hydronephrosis indicated by stretching of arteries. Fine neovascularity and staining throughout kidney compatible with xanthogranulomatous pyelonephritis

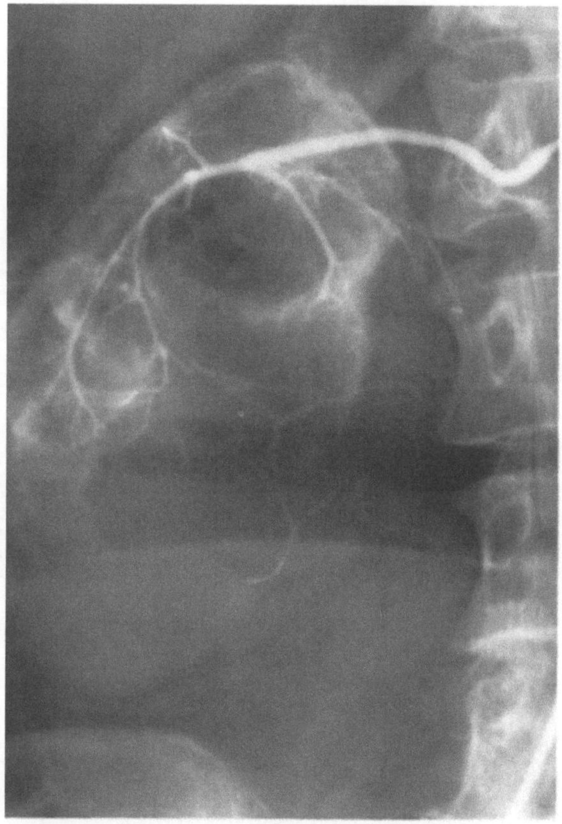

Fig. 12C

It is in these cases where painstaking comparison of ultrasound, urographic, and puncture findings are particularly important if the tumor is to be recognized. Fortunately, tumor within a cyst is quite rare (LANG, 1971c; SILVERMAN and KILHENNY, 1969; WEITZNER, 1971; GROSS and BEACH, 1971).

HOLM et al. (1972b) has pointed out the difficulty in diagnosing transitional cell carcinoma of the renal pelvis by ultrasound. Because of the homogenous nature of such tumors, they frequently simulate cystic lesions (Fig. 14). From a practical clinical standpoint this is not of great importance since the urographic features of renal pelvis carcinoma and central renal cysts are quite different. Here again, careful comparison of urographic and ultrasonographic data will prevent diagnostic errors.

It should be clearly stated that ultrasound is not appropriate as a screening procedure to *detect* renal masses. Small- or moderate-sized solid lesions can easily blend in with the renal parenchyma, especially

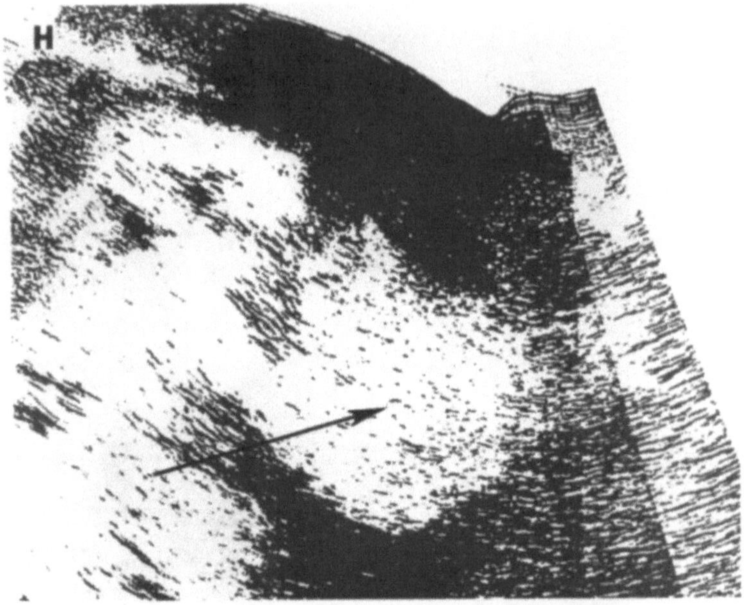

A

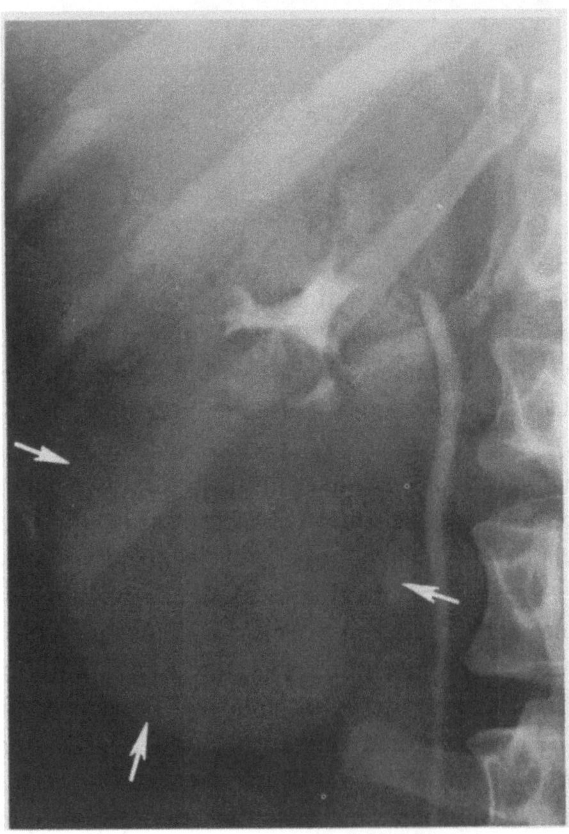

Fig. 13A and B B

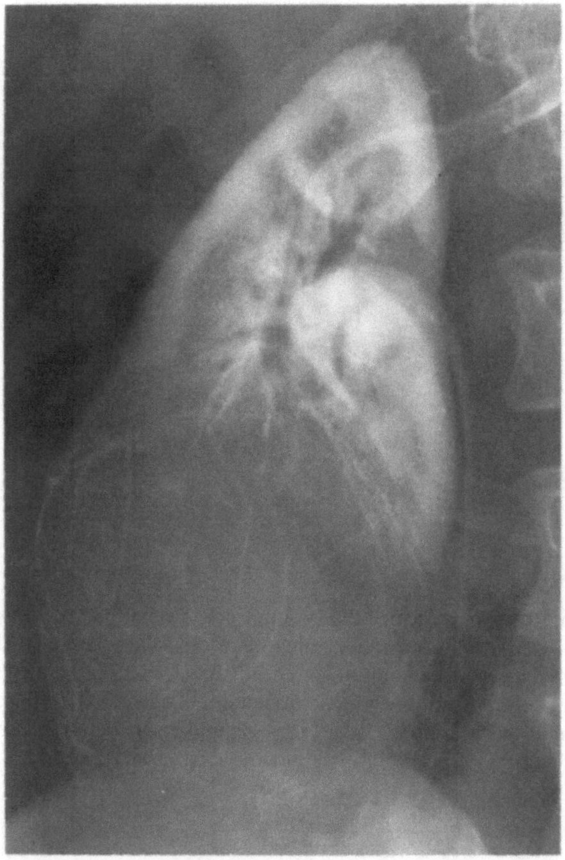

Fig. 13C

Fig. 13. (A) Prone, longitudinal scan. Renal fibroma. Solid mass replaces right lower pole. Specific diagnosis not possible. (B) Excretory urogram. Large lower pole mass *(arrows)* produces marked caliceal compression. (C) Renal arteriogram, nephrographic phase. Modest tumor vascularity present. Determination of benign versus malignant tumor cannot be made

if they are deep-seated masses without renal contour deformity. When the intravenous urogram merely raises the suspicion of a renal mass, nephrotomography should be carried out. When a mass is documented by nephrotomography, ultrasonic scanning can then be done to determine its consistency.

II. Renal Biopsy

Since the ultrasonic scans allow precise determination of kidney position relative to the overlying flank, its use has been advocated in the

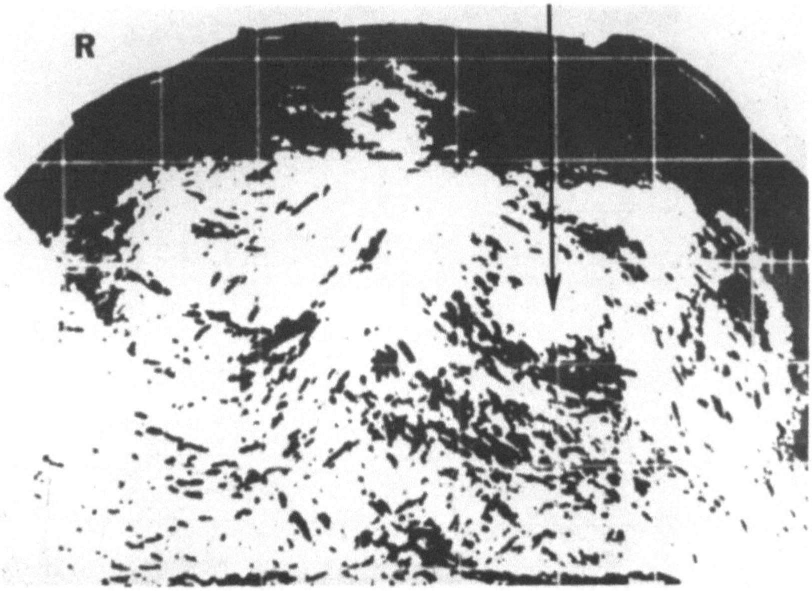

A

Fig. 14. (A) Prone, transverse scan. Transitional cell carcinoma, left renal pelvis. *Arrow* points to center of nearly echo-free mass which displaces calices laterally. (B) Nephrotomogram. Large mass invades and amputates entire upper pole collecting system. (C) Left renal arteriogram, left posterior oblique projection. Transitional cell carcinoma causes separation and smooth encasement of arteries around renal pelvis. Characteristic hypertrophy of pelvic branches of the renal artery *(arrow)*.

performance of percutaneous renal biopsy (KRISTENSEN et al., 1972; MAXWELL and ASHER, 1974). Care should be taken to mark the puncture site on the skin in the same phase of respiration in which biopsy will be performed.

Although the biopsy transducer has also been recommended for this procedure, the borders of the kidney are usually harder to discern on the A-mode display since no fluid-filled spaces are involved.

III. Perirenal Fluid Collections

Because of its unique ability to define even small fluid collections, ultrasonic scanning has proved to be extremely useful in the identification of a wide variety of disorders of the perirenal spaces (LEOPOLD and ASHER, 1972; LEOPOLD, 1973). Hemorrhage, abscess, and urinoma can all be nicely demonstrated, although differentiation among them is usually not possible without clinical history. It is frequently possible

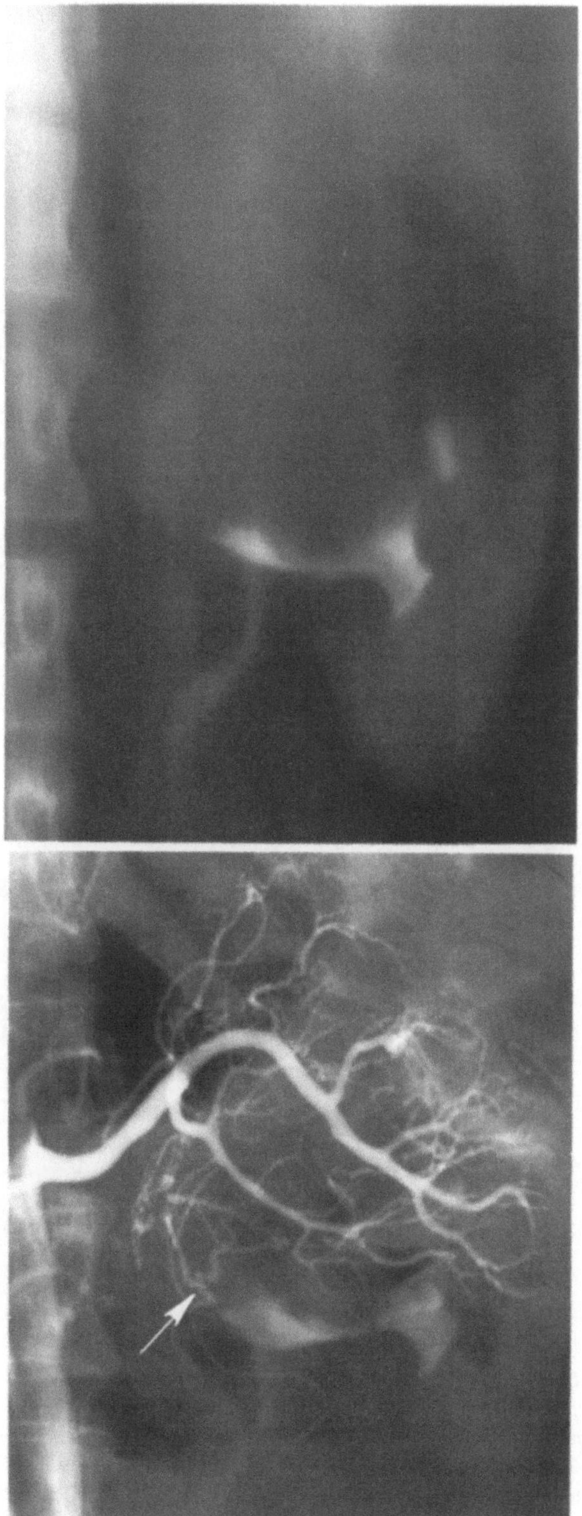

B

C

Fig. 14B and C

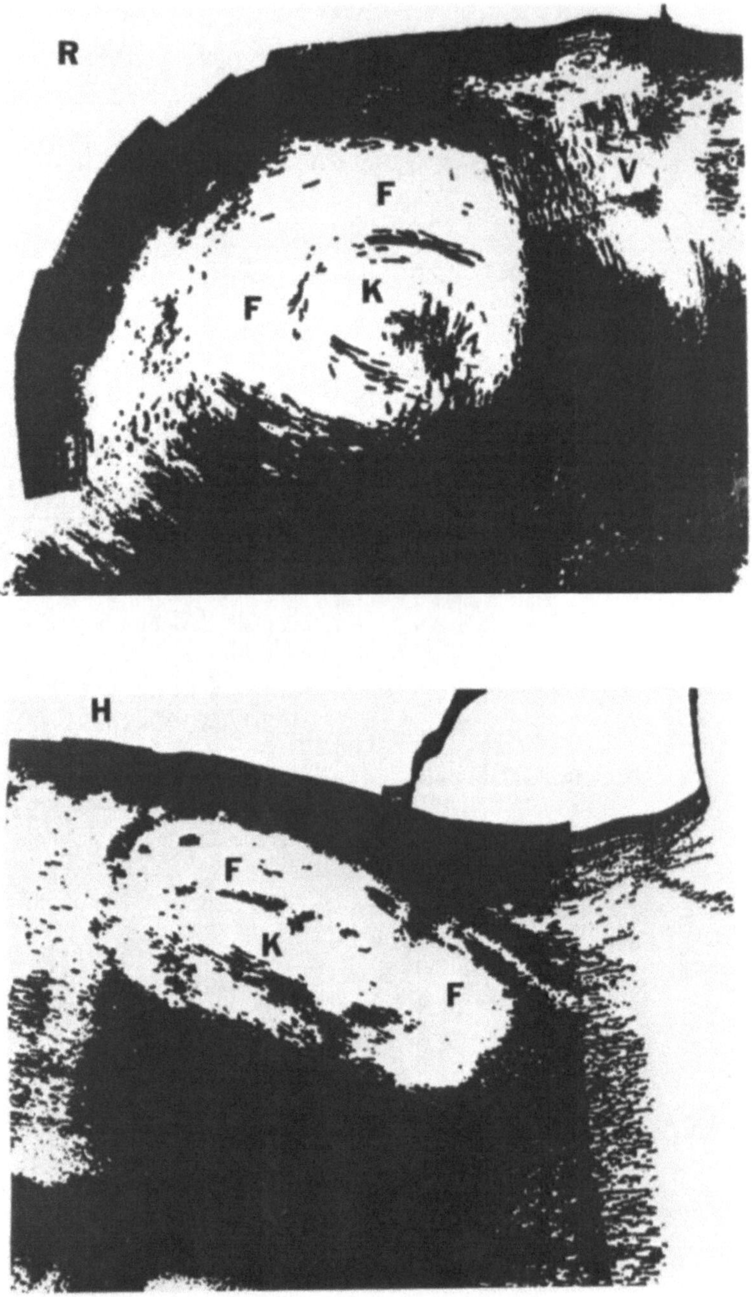

A

B

Fig. 15. (A) Prone, transverse scan. Perirenal urinoma and hematoma from penetrating injury. Fluid (*F*) within perirenal space appears sonolucent. Renal capsule separates extrarenal fluid from kidney parenchyma (*K*). *V*=vertebral column. (B) Prone, longitudinal scan. Relationship between perirenal fluid (*F*) and renal parenchyma (*K*) confirmed in sagittal plane. (C) Excretory urogram. Contrast material extravasates from collecting system into perirenal space.

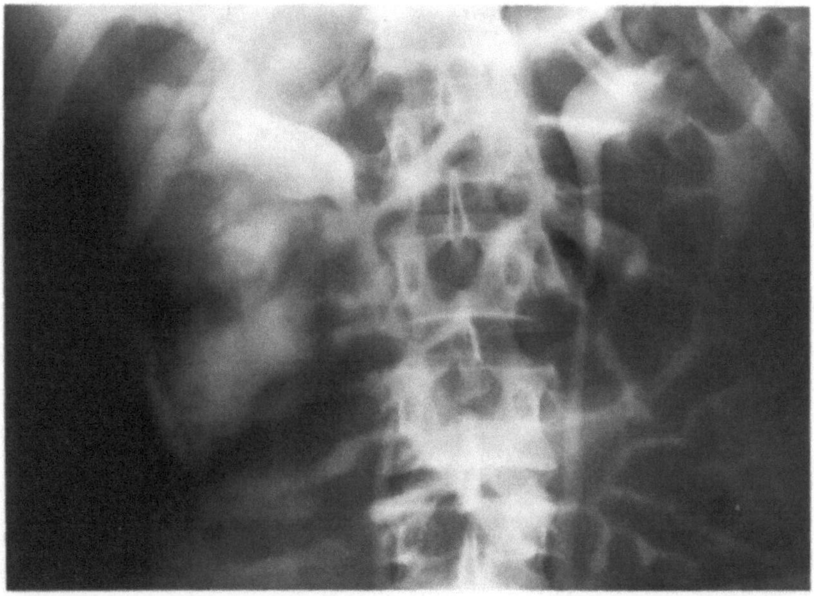

Fig. 15C

to predict which retroperitoneal compartment is involved based on the ultrasonic localization of the fluid. Collections posterior to the kidney in all scans are usually located behind the posterior leaf of Gerota's fascia. If the collection surrounds the kidney anteriorly and posteriorly, it almost surely lies within Gerota's fascia (Fig. 15). The predominant accumulation of fluid will be lateral, inferior, and slightly posterior to the kidney since this fat-containing region represents the greatest potential space. A localized collection of fluid immediately adjacent to the kidney, associated with compression of the calices, suggests a subcapsular accumulation (Fig. 16). This is particularly apt to occur with spontaneous hemorrhage or hemorrhage related to trauma. It is not unusual in this situation for the kidney to be nonfunctioning on urography (KOEHLER et al., 1973).

If the collection is anterior and medial to the kidney, origin from one of the structures lying between the anterior leaf of Gerota's fascia and the posterior peritoneum (pancreas, duodenum, colon) is likely.

In view of the high morbidity and mortality which results from undiagnosed retroperitoneal abscess and the frequent difficulty in demonstrating such lesions by radiographic and angiographic techniques, ultrasonic scanning has proved a very welcome diagnostic addition (Fig. 17).

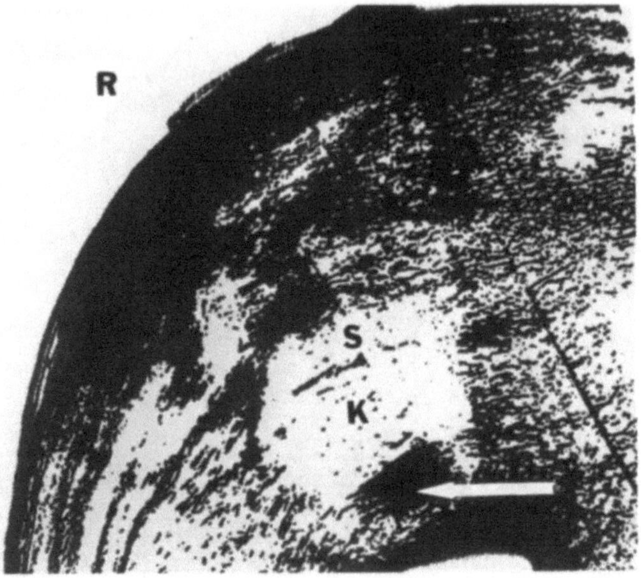

A

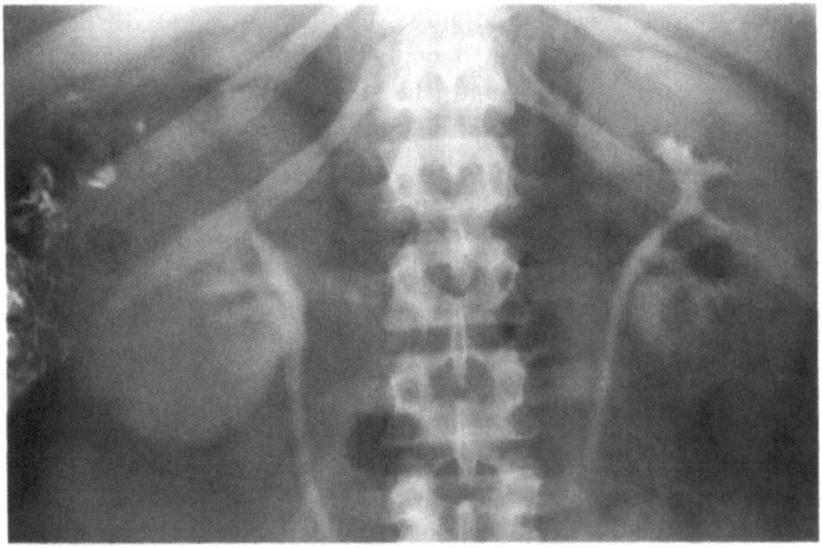

B

Fig. 16. (A) Prone, transverse scan. Subcapsular (*S*) and intraparenchymal (*K*) hematoma from penetrating trauma. Medial displacement of the calices *(arrow)*. (B) Excretory urogram. Increased tissue pressure from subcapsular collection causes compression and poor filling of calices on right. Residual barium in ascending colon

IV. Perirenal Masses

Ultrasonic analysis has been helpful in the evaluation of many solid masses which occur near the renal fossa, including enlarged retroperitoneal lymph nodes and primary retroperitoneal tumors (SMITH and BARTRUM, 1975; HOLM et al., 1972a). Scans help in documenting the response to treatment as well as in planning the actual treatment portals if radiation therapy is employed. By directly transposing the ultrasonic cross-sectional anatomy of the tumor to the patient's contour, the radiation therapist greatly improves the accuracy of his dosimetry to both the tumor and surrounding normal structures.

Adrenal lesions are usually visualized slightly anterior to the upper pole of the kidney and are easiest to recognize in sagittal projection (Fig. 18). The ultrasonic appearance of adrenal masses is much less characteristic than that of renal masses. Adrenal cysts frequently contain hemorrhagic debris which generates multiple internal echoes, thereby simulating a complex or solid lesion. Calcification in the wall of such cysts may cause reverberation echoes, again producing a solid appearance. In most cases, adrenal lesions can be separated from upper pole renal lesions on sagittal scans. However, when an adrenal tumor has invaded the kidney parenchyma, differentiation from a primary renal tumor is impossible solely on the basis of the ultrasonic scan. In these cases angiography may similarly fail to make this distinction.

Ultrasound has been useful to the authors in the evaluation of patients with suspected pheochromocytoma, especially when the tumors are multiple or in extra-adrenal sites.

V. Hydronephrosis

Early in the course of obstructive uropathy, sufficient dilatation of the renal pelvis occurs to produce a recognizable ultrasonic pattern (KYLE et al., 1971) (Fig. 19). The normally dense cluster of caliceal echoes assumes a rounded- or O-shaped configuration with a central clear space, first described by BARNETT and MORLEY (1971). While this is usually a very helpful sign, confusion sometimes arises in the presence of a large extrarenal pelvis, peripelvic cyst, or extensive renal sinus lipomatosis (Fig. 9).

As the duration and degree of hydronephrosis increases, the central clear space becomes even more striking and easier to recognize. If ante-

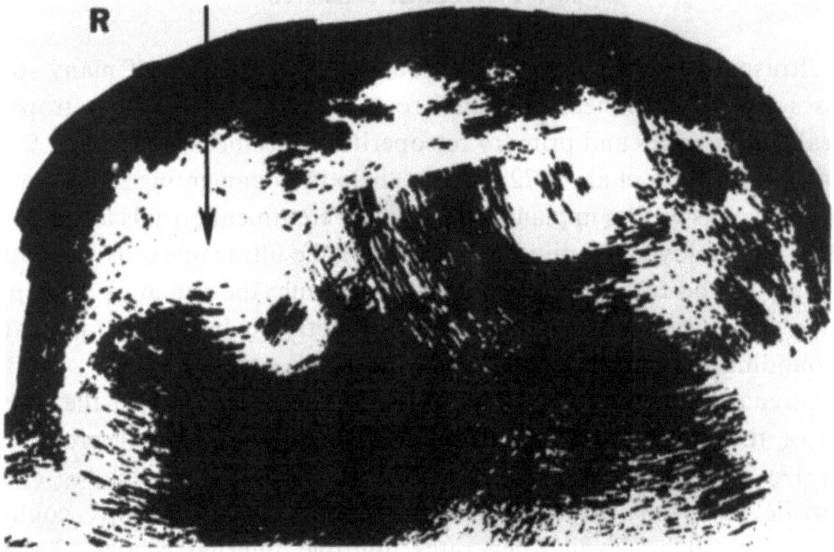

A

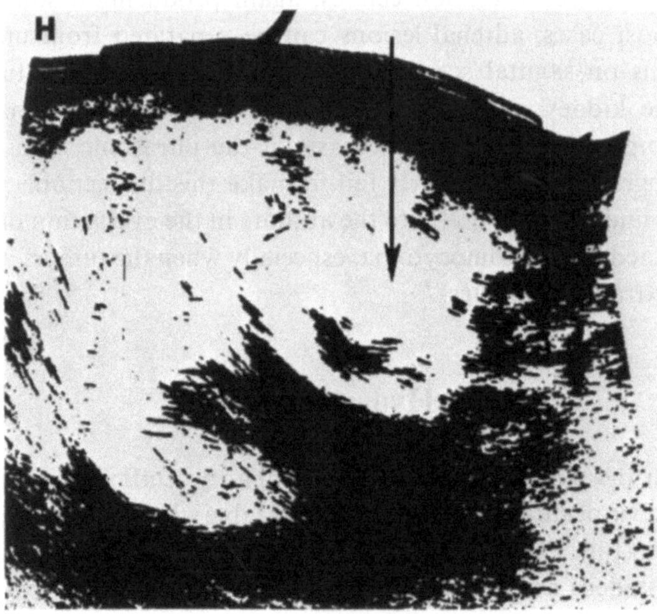

B

Fig. 17. (A) Prone, transverse scan. Right perinephric abscess in diabetic patient with papillary necrosis. Irregular mass *(arrow)* behind kidney pushes entire kidney forward. Scattered internal echoes indicate complex nature of mass. (B) Prone, longitudinal scan. Sagittal display confirms appearance in A. Some caliceal compression due to associated intrarenal renal abscess. Note liver edge anterior to kidney. (C) Excretory urogram. Poor filling of right lower pole calices and loss of renal outline indicates intrarenal involvement but gives little evidence of extensive perirenal collection. Latter is best shown by ultrasound

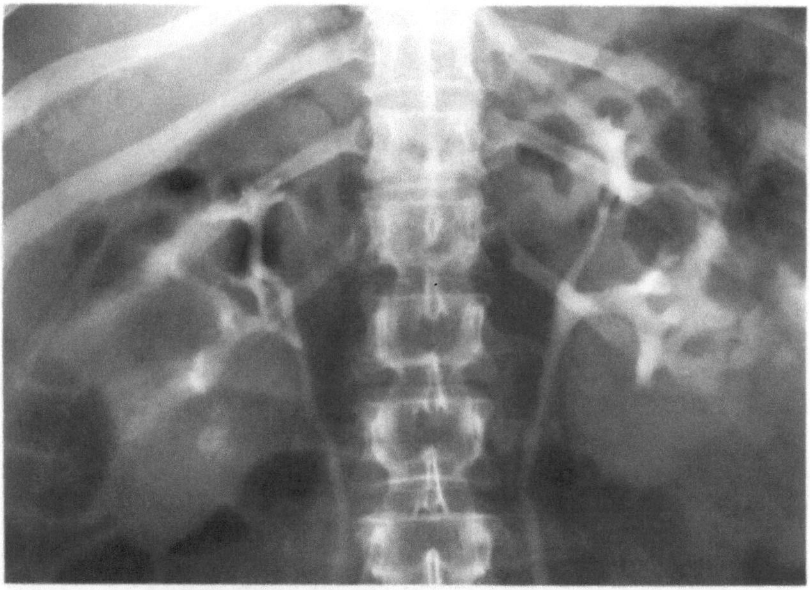

Fig. 17C

grade pyelography is desired to characterize the nature of the obstruction, spatial information obtained from the ultrasonic scan may be useful in percutaneous insertion of the needle (PEDERSEN, 1974) (Fig. 19C).

In end stage hydronephrosis the renal fossa is filled with a large fluid-containing sac that has few or absent internal echoes. While this pattern is most striking in adults with long-standing ureteropelvic junction obstruction (SANDERS and BEARMAN, 1973), it can be easily shown in newborn infants and children as well (LYONS et al., 1972; HASCH, 1974) (Fig. 20). Because it gives an answer within minutes and is noninvasive, a case can be made for using ultrasound early in the evaluation of newborn infants with renal failure or large abdominal masses. Intravenous urography may yield similar information, but has the disadvantage that delayed films may be needed before treatment can be instituted. On the other hand, ultrasonic demonstration of two normal kidneys and collecting systems may obviate the need for emergency uroradiologic study.

VI. Renal Transplants

Since the usual site for transplantation in adults is into the iliac fossa, a relatively superficial area, the kidney is even more accessible

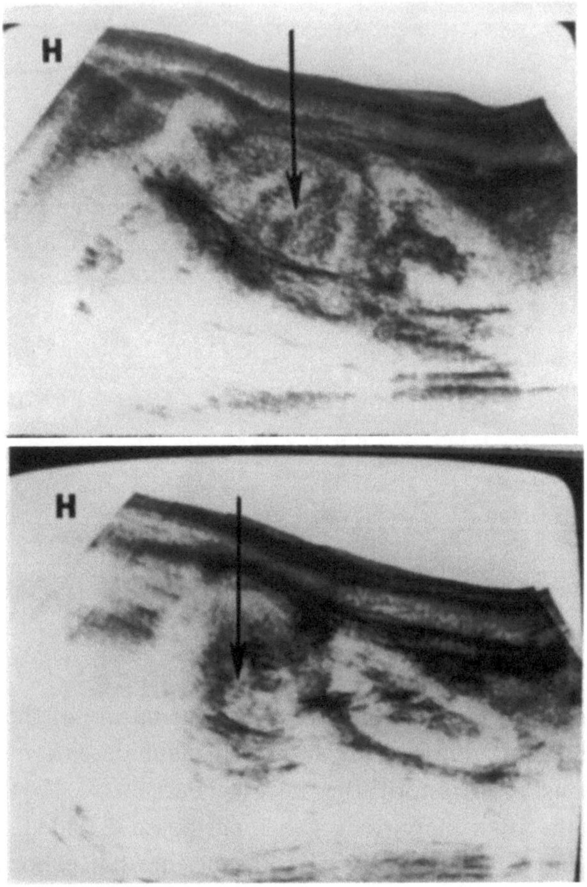

Figs. 18A and B. Prone, longitudinal scans (gray scale). Bilateral adrenal metastases from oat cell carcinoma of lung. *Arrows* point to center of solid adrenal masses on left (A) and right (B). Clearcut separation of mass from kidney indicates extrarenal origin. (C) Excretory urogram. Flattening of right upper pole and distortion of both renal axes from adrenal masses

to ultrasonic scanning than in its normal location (LEOPOLD, 1970; WINTERBERGER et al., 1972). Longitudinal scans delineate the entire kidney as well as the iliopsoas muscle on which it rests (Fig. 21A). By taking multiple transverse sections and noting the position of the central caliceal pattern on each, it is possible to perform a sagittal scan exactly along the longitudinal axis of the kidney. Precise measurements of transplant size can be used to evaluate rejection, particularly if performed on a serial basis. This method is superior to the usual radiographic methods for measuring transplant size, since the latter involve magnification factors which may be quite different for each end of the kidney.

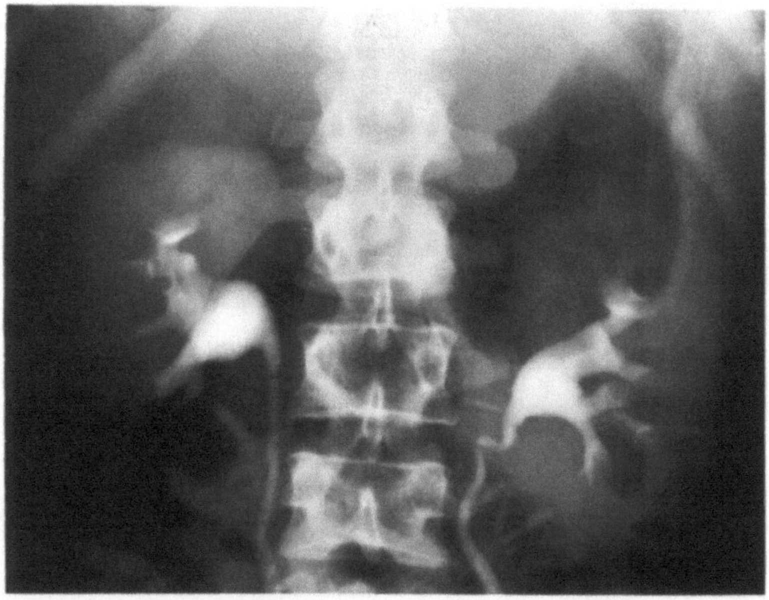

Fig. 18C

Some authors, in an effort to approach the problem more quantitatively, have advocated serial ultrasonic sections through the kidney with planigraphic area determination of each section (BARTRUM et al., 1974). The individual areas are integrated to give an estimated renal volume which has proved to be highly accurate.

In addition to rejection, other major complications of renal transplantation may also be apparent on ultrasonic scans. Obstruction of the transplant ureter leads to changes in the collecting system echo pattern identical to those in the obstructed, but normally situated, kidney. Fluid collections around the transplant may be due to urinoma (Fig. 21B), abscess, retroperitoneal hemorrhage, or occasionally, lymphocele (RASHID et al., 1974; SCHWEIZER et al., 1972). Since each of these complications requires a specific treatment different from the more common rejection reaction, ultrasonic scanning has become an important step in early evaluation of declining urinary output following transplantation.

VII. Urinary Bladder

1. Bladder Volumes

Since the urinary bladder is usually fluid filled and lies anteriorly, it is quite simple to examine ultrasonically. A series of transverse and

A

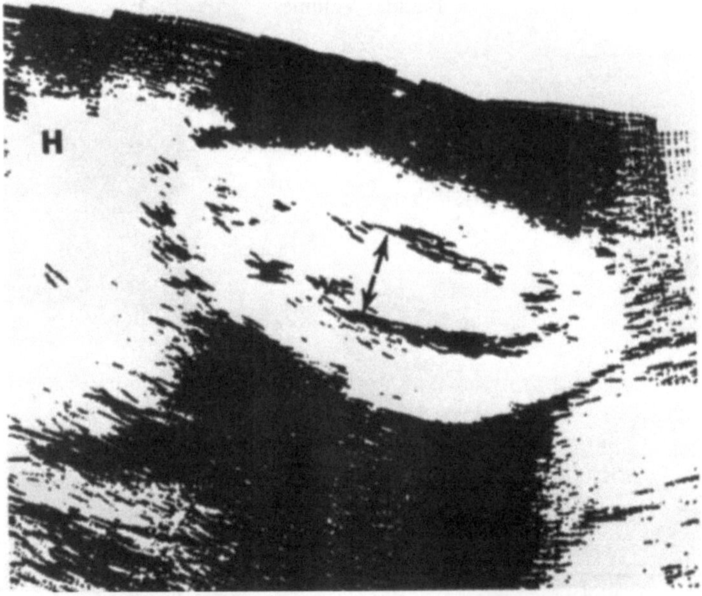

B

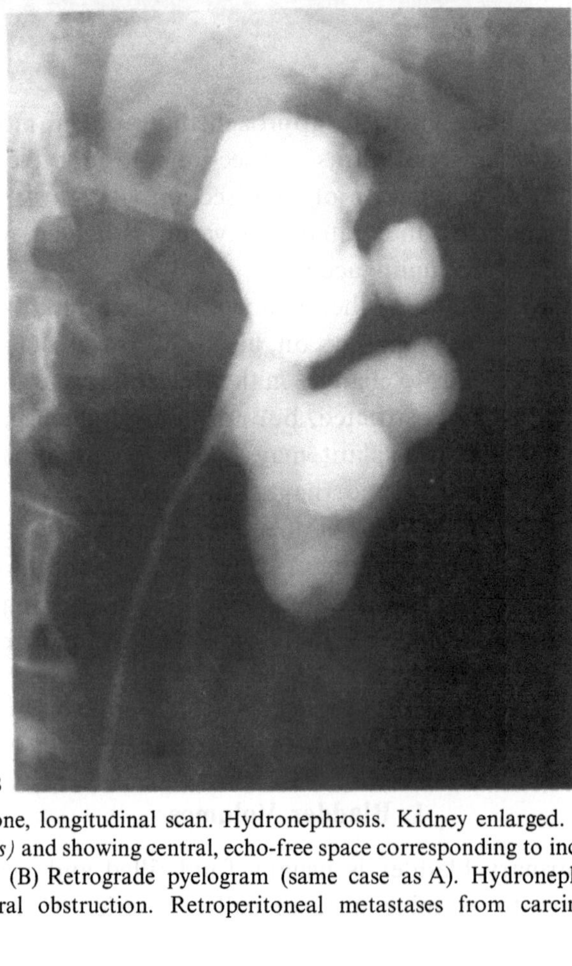

Fig. 19. (A) Prone, longitudinal scan. Hydronephrosis. Kidney enlarged. Caliceal margins widened *(arrows)* and showing central, echo-free space corresponding to increased collecting system volume. (B) Retrograde pyelogram (same case as A). Hydronephrosis caused by proximal ureteral obstruction. Retroperitoneal metastases from carcinoma of breast.

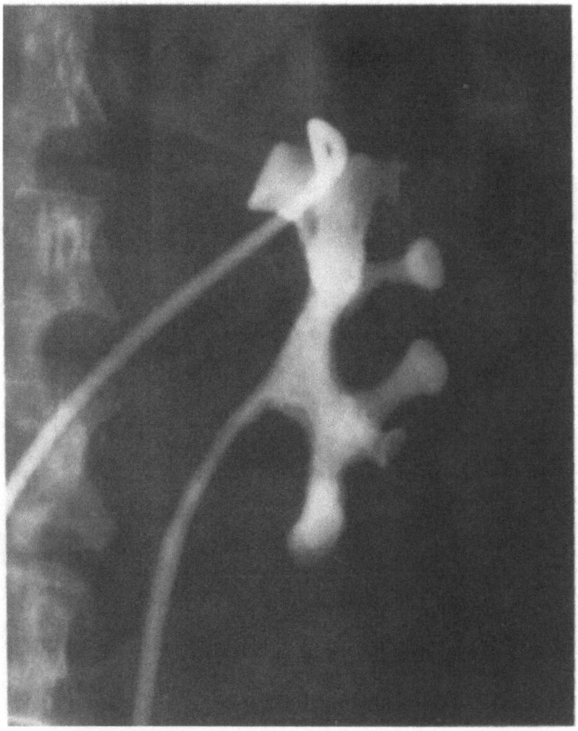

C

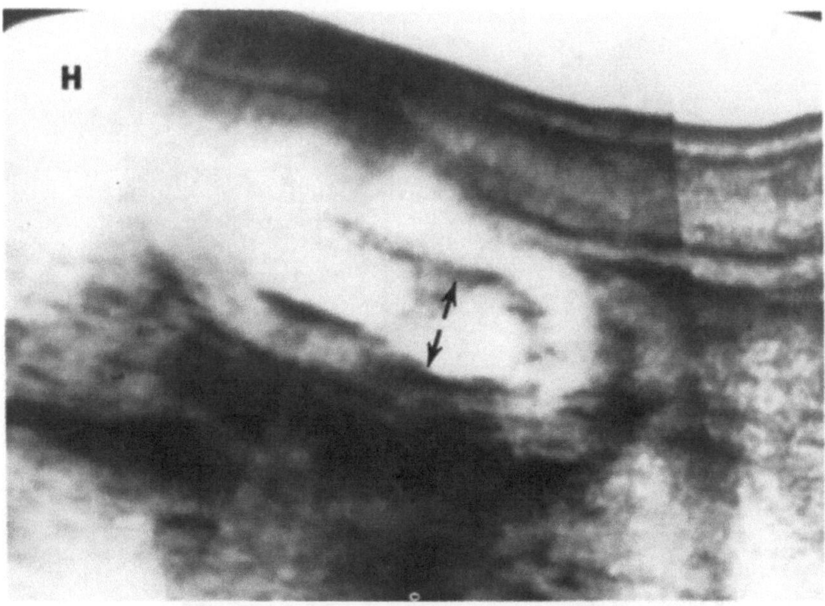

D

(C) Nephrostomy tube injection (same case as A and B). Decompression of hydronephrosis accomplished by percutaneous nephrostomy using ultrasound guidance. (D) Prone, transverse scan (gray scale). Hydronephrosis of pregnancy, right kidney. Gray scale facilitates distinction between renal parenchyma and collecting system. Caliceal margins widened *(arrows)* similar to A

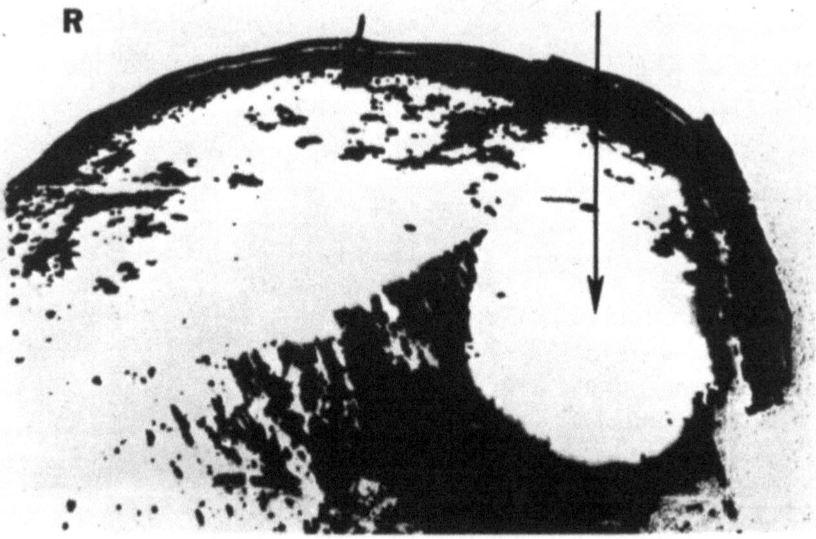

A

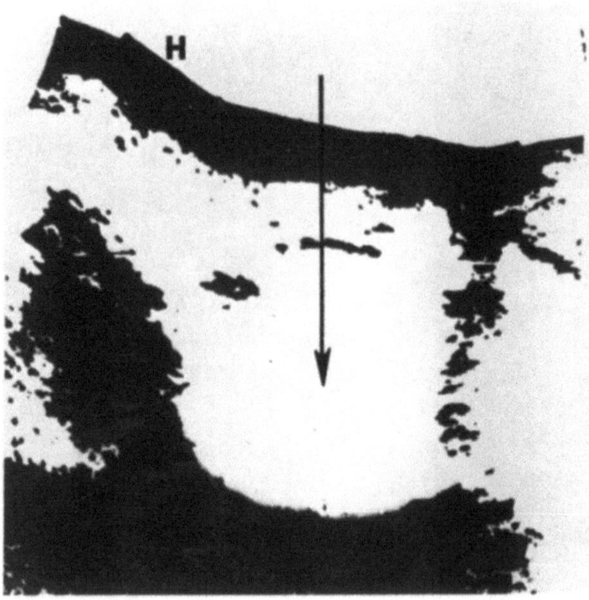

B

Fig. 20. (A) Prone, transverse scan. Congenital uretero-pelvic junction obstruction in a child. Massively dilated left renal pelvis *(arrow)*. (B) Prone, longitudinal scan. Renal pelvis *(arrow)* projects anteriorly and corresponds to findings in A. Compressed renal parenchyma posteriorly

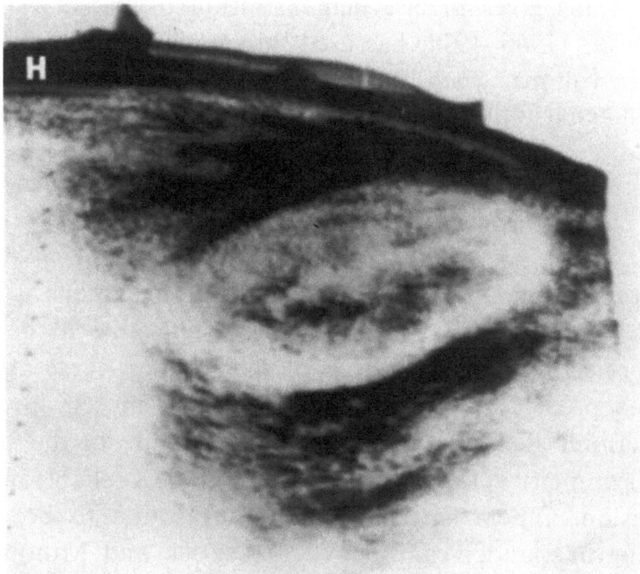

A

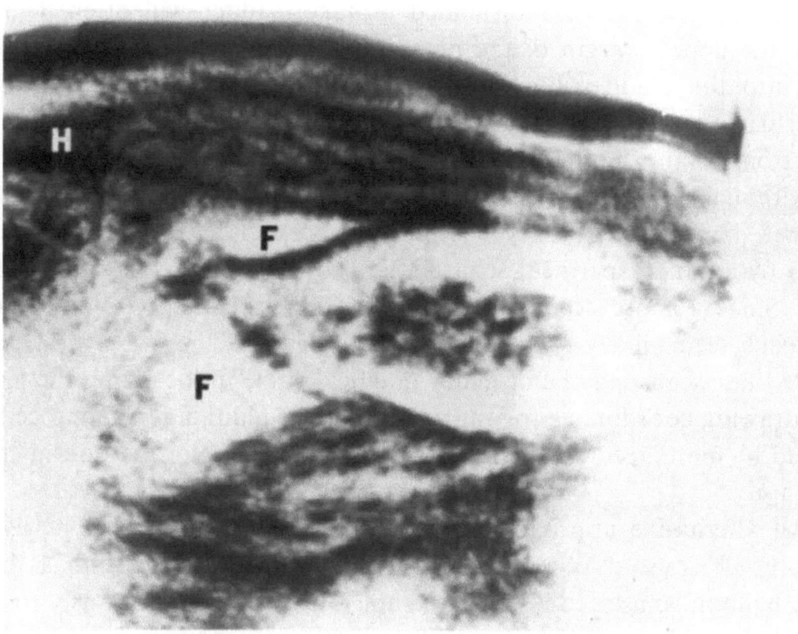

B

Fig. 21. (A) Supine, longitudinal scan (gray scale). Normal renal transplant in iliac fossa. Note superficial location of kidney. (B) Supine, longitudinal scan. Extravasation of urine from renal transplant. Fluid collection (*F*) surrounds upper pole of kidney longitudinal scans gives precise demonstration of the margins of the bladder. HOLMES (1966, 1971) has used this noninvasive method to estimate bladder volume. Such measurements have been used to follow patients with renal failure where the introduction of a catheter might be hazardous.

2. Bladder Tumors

BARNETT and MORLEY (1971) have found the technique to be useful in studying vesical tumors. In addition to being able to demonstrate the tumor projecting into the lumen of the bladder, these authors feel that they can predict the presence or absence of muscle invasion and thereby determine the stage of such lesions. Failure of the bladder to distend in a symmetrical fashion is considered to be a reliable indicator of muscle invasion. Others have not found ultrasound to be as helpful in the staging of bladder cancer (WINTERBERGER and MURPHY, 1974).

3. Prostatic Scanning

Careful scanning of a distended urinary bladder will often demonstrate the upper margin of the prostate which, if enlarged, may project well into the bladder lumen (MILLER et al., 1972) (Fig. 22). This is particularly true of median bar hypertrophy which may be difficult to detect on rectal examination.

Although a rough estimate of gland size may be obtained in this manner, improved accuracy has recently been claimed (WENZEL et al., 1974) by adding a perineal scan to the ordinary supine, sagittal, pelvic scan. Since a more complete outline of the prostate is obtained, this approach seems likely to gain in popularity.

Prostate scans may be of major practical value in localizing the gland and drawing coordinates for radiation therapy planning. This procedure should be more accurate than the mercury bag-catheter method in common use.

An alternative approach to prostatic scanning has been suggested recently (WATANABE et al., 1974). An ultrasonic probe within a fluid-filled balloon is inserted into the rectum. The probe continuously rotates a full 360°, giving a circular view of the prostate and base of the bladder. Preliminary work with this instrument suggests that it may afford an even more accurate assessment of prostatic volume than the previously described methods. Although it is usually possible to distinguish prostatic

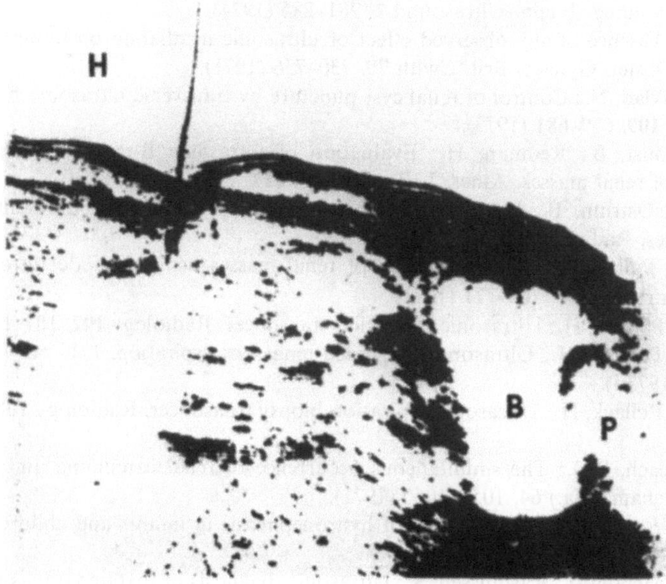

Fig. 22. Supine, longitudinal scan. Prostatic hypertrophy. Enlarged prostate gland (*P*) bulges into base of urine filled bladder (*B*)

nodules from normal gland, the distinction between malignant and benign prostatic nodules is not yet a reality.

Summary

While the use of ultrasonic scanning is still in its infancy, the authors firmly believe that the future will witness an expansion of indications as instrumentation and anatomic detail continue to improve. It seems certain that urologists and radiologists can look forward with justifiable optimism to the next series of developments in urinary tract ultrasound.

References

Asher, W., Leopold, G.: A streamlined approach to renal mass lesions with renal echograms. J. Urol. (Baltimore) **108**, 205–209 (1972).

Barnett, E., Morley, P.: Ultrasound in the diagnosis of space occupying lesions of the urinary tract. Brit. J. Radiol. **44**, 733–742 (1971).

Bartrum, R., Smith, E., D'Orsi, C., Dantono, J.: The ultrasonic determination of renal transplant volume. J. clin. Ultrasound **2**, 281–285 (1974).
Bobrow, M.: Absence of any observed effect of ultrasonic irradiation on human chromosomes. J. Obstet. Gynaec. Brit. Cwlth **78**, 730–736 (1971).
Doust, B., Maklad, N.: Control of renal cyst puncture by transverse ultrasonic B-scanning. Radiology **109**, 679–681 (1973).
Doust, V., Doust, B., Redman, H.: Evaluation of ultrasonic B-mode scanning in the diagnosis of renal masses. Amer. J. Roentgenol. **117**, 112–118 (1973).
Goldberg, B., Ostrum, B., Isard, H.: Nephrosonography: ultrasound differentiation of renal masses. Radiology **90**, 1113–1118 (1968).
Goldberg, B., Pollack, H.: Differentiation of renal masses using A-mode ultrasound. J. Urol. (Baltimore) **105**, 765–771 (1971).
Goldberg, B., Pollack, H.: Ultrasonic aspiration transducer. Radiology **102**, 187–189 (1972).
Goldberg, B., Pollack, H.: Ultrasonically guided renal cyst aspiration. J. Urol. (Baltimore) **109**, 5–7 (1973a).
Goldberg, B., Pollack, H.: Ultrasonic aspiration-biopsy transducer. Radiology **108**, 667–671 (1973b).
Gross, M., Beach, P.D.: The simultaneous occurrence of renal carcinoma and cyst. Sth. med. J. (Bgham, Ala.) **64**, 1059–1060 (1971).
Hasch, E.: Ultrasound in the diagnosis of hydronephrosis in infants and children. J. clin. Ultrasound **2**, 21–25 (1974).
Holm, H., Kristensen, J., Rasmussen, S.: Ultrasonic diagnosis of juxtarenal masses. Scand. J. Urol. Nephrol. (Suppl. 15) **6**, 83–89 (1972a).
Holm, H., Rasmussen, S., Kristensen, J.: Errors and pitfalls in ultrasonic scanning of the abdomen. Brit. J. Radiol. **45**, 835–840 (1972b).
Holmes, J.: Diagnostic study of the abdomen. In: Ultrasonographia Medica, Vol. III. Wien: Verlag der Wiener Medizinischen Akademie 1971.
Holmes, J.: Ultrasonic studies of the bladder and kidney. In: Diagnostic Ultrasound. New York: Plenum Press 1966.
Jeans, W.D., Penry, J.B., Roylance, J.: Renal puncture. Clin. Radiol. **23**, 298–311 (1972).
King, D.: Renal ultrasonography. Radiology **105**, 633–640 (1972).
Koehler, P., Talner, L., Friedenberg, M., Kyaw, M.: Association of subcapsular hematomas with the nonfunctioning kidney. Radiology **106**, 537–542 (1973).
Kristensen, J., Bartels, E., Jorgensen, H.: Percutaneous renal biopsy under the guidance of ultrasound. Scand. J. Urol. Nephrol. **8**, 223–226 (1974).
Kristensen, J., Holm, H., Rasmussen, S., Barlebo, H.: Ultrasonically guided percutaneous puncture of renal masses. Scand. J. Urol. Nephrol. (Suppl. 15) **6**, 49–56 (1972).
Kyle, K., Deane, R., Morley, P., Barnett, E.: Ultrasonography of the urinary tract. Brit. J. Urol. **43**, 709–717 (1971).
Lalli, A.: Percutaneous aspiration of renal masses. Amer. J. Roentgenol. **101**, 700–704 (1967).
Lang, E.K.: The differential diagnosis of renal cysts and tumors. Radiology **87**, 883–888 (1966).
Lang, E.K.: The accuracy of roentgenographic techniques in the diagnosis of renal mass lesions. Radiology **98**, 119–128 (1971a).
Lang, E.K.: The roentgenographic diagnosis of renal mass lesions. St. Louis: Warren H. Green, Inc. 1971b.
Lang, E.K.: Coexistence of cyst and tumor in the same kidney. Radiology **101**, 7–16 (1971c).
Lang, E.K.: Roentgenographic assessment of asymptomatic renal lesions. Radiology **109**, 257–269 (1973).

Leopold, G.: Renal transplant size measured by reflected ultrasound. Radiology **95**, 687–689 (1970).

Leopold, G.: A review of retroperitoneal ultrasonography. J. clin. Ultrasound **1**, 82–87 (1973).

Leopold, G., Asher, W.: Diagnosis of extra-organ retroperitoneal space lesions by B-scan ultrasonography. Radiology **104**, 133–138 (1972).

Leopold, G., Talner, L., Asher, W., Gosink, B., Gittes, R.: Renal echography: an updated approach to the diagnosis of renal cyst. Radiology **109**, 671–678 (1973).

Lindblom, K.: Diagnostic kidney puncture of cysts and tumors. Amer. J. Roentgenol. **68**, 209–215 (1952).

Lyons, E., Murphy, A., Arneil, G.: Sonar and its use in kidney disease in children. Arch. Dis. Childh. **47**, 777–786 (1972).

Maxwell, D., Asher, W.: Ultrasound localization of the kidneys for closed renal biopsies. J. clin. Ultrasound **2**, 279–280 (1974).

McLaughlin, A.P., Talner, L.B., Leopold, G.R., McCullough, D.L.: Avascular primary renal cell carcinoma; Varied pathologic and angiographic features. J. Urol. (Baltimore) **111**, 587–593 (1974).

Miller, S., Christie, A., Smith, G.: Evaluation of prostatic disease by ultrasound. Brit. J. Surg. **59**, 302–303 (1972).

Mountford, R., Ross, F., Burwood, R.: The use of ultrasound in the diagnosis of renal disease. Brit. J. Radiol. **44**, 860–869 (1971).

Olsson, O.: Roentgendiagnosis of the kidney and the ureter. Berlin-Heidelberg-New York: Springer 1973.

Pedersen, J.: Percutaneous nephrostomy guided by ultrasound. J. Urol. (Baltimore) **112**, 157–159 (1974).

Rashid, A., Posen, G., Couture, R., McKay, D., Wellington, J.: Accumulation of lymph around the transplanted kidney (lymphocele) mimicking renal allograft rejection. J. Urol. (Baltimore) **111**, 145–147 (1974).

Romeiser, R., Walls, W., Valk, W.: B-scan ultrasound in the evaluation of renal mass lesions. J. Urol. (Baltimore) **112**, 8–12 (1974).

Sanders, R.C., Bearman, S.: B-scan ultrasound in the diagnosis of hydronephrosis. Radiology **108**, 375–382 (1973).

Schreck, W., Holmes, J.: Ultrasound as a diagnostic aid for renal neoplasms and cysts. J. Urol. (Baltimore) **103**, 281–285 (1970).

Schreeb, T. von, Franzen, S., Ljungqvist, A.: Renal adenocarcinoma: evaluation of malignancy on a cytologic basis: a comparative cytologic and histologic study. Scand. J. Urol. Nephrol. **1**, 265–269 (1967).

Schweizer, R., Sang-In, C., Kountz, S., Belzer, F.: Lymphoceles following renal transplantation. Arch. Surg. **104**, 40–45 (1972).

Sherwood, T., Stevenson, J.J.: Management of renal masses. Clin. Radiol. **22**, 180–187 (1971).

Silverman, J.F., Kilhenny, C.: Tumor in the wall of a simple renal cyst. Radiology **93**, 95–98 (1969).

Smith, E., Bartrum, R.: Ultrasonic evaluation of pararenal masses. J. Amer. med. Ass. **231**, 51–55 (1975).

Smith, E., Bennett, A.: The usefulness of ultrasound in the evaluation of renal masses in adults. J. Urol. (Baltimore) **113**, 525–530 (1975).

Steg, A., Boccon-Gibod, L., Charles, J.F., Aboulker, P.: La ponction percutanée dans le diagnostic des tumeurs du rein. Ann. Urol. **5**, 203–213 (1971).

Stuber, J., Templeton, A., Bishop, K.: Ultrasonic evaluation of the kidneys. Radiology **104**, 139–143 (1972).

Thornbury, J.R.: Needle aspiration of avascular renal lesions. Radiology **105**, 299–302 (1972).

Watanabe, H., Igari, D., Tanahasi, Y., Harada, K., Saitoh, M.: Development and application of new equipment for transrectal ultrasonography. J. clin. Ultrasound **2**, 91–98 (1974).

Weitzner, S.: Clear cell carcinoma of the free wall of a renal cyst. J. Urol. (Baltimore) **106**, 515–517 (1971).

Wenzel, W., Johnson, F., Carson, P.: Prostate localization using ultrasound B-mode scanning. Presented at 19th AIUM meeting, October 5–10, Seattle, Wash. 1974.

Winterberger, A., Palma, L., Murphy, G.: Ultrasonic testing in human renal allografts. J. Amer. med. Ass. **219**, 475–479 (1972).

Winterberger, A.R., Murphy, G.P.: Correlation of B-scan ultrasonic laminography with bilateral selective hypogastric arteriography and lymphography in bladder tumors. Vasc. Surg. **8**, 169–176 (1974).

Percutaneous Puncture Nephrostomy

By

I. Fernström and L. Andersson

With 30 Figures

A. Introduction

In recent years temporary nephrostomy or pyelostomy has increasingly been used to preserve renal function in cases of ureteric obstruction or injury, in which primary ureteric surgery is considered injudicious or impossible. Such is the case if the lower ureter is injured during a hysterectomy or rectal amputation, if suture lines of ileal conduits and ureterosigmoidostomies leak, or if ureteric suture lines swell and obstruct. An infected kidney which is excluded not only fails very rapidly, but also constitutes a major risk for general septicemia, and immediate drainage is imperative. These and other situations, for which temporary, or perhaps even permanent, nephrostomy is indicated, will subsequently be discussed more fully.

B. Operative Nephrostomy

Performance of a nephrostomy or pyelostomy is a well-established procedure in which the kidney is usually reached by a lumbar approach. In cases of recent obstruction the operation is usually simple, but when there has been an obstruction of longer duration, fibrosis and adhesions may add considerably to the operative difficulties. The pelvis, usually opened on the dorsal side, is dissected free from the renal vessels, and the pyelostomy or nephrostomy catheter is introduced. In spite of a somewhat increased bleeding risk, a nephrostomy is preferable to a pyelostomy, for there is less leakage, less risk of the catheter falling out, and a more comfortable location laterally on the abdominal wall than in a pyelostomy using the dorsal approach.

Since operative nephrostomy carries the risks of any comparable kidney operation, it must be considered a major procedure when performed on patients debilitated by chronic illness, previous surgery, or both.

C. Percutaneous Puncture of the Renal Pelvis

With the development of percutaneous puncture of the renal pelvis for antegrade pyelo-ureterography in the 1950's and later, there arose the idea of renal drainage by a similar technique (WICKBOM, 1954; GOODWIN *et al.*, 1955; BARTLEY *et al.*, 1965; MOLIN and ULMSTEN, 1971; VELA NAVARRETE, 1971; JONSSON *et al.*, 1972; ULMSTEN and MOLIN, 1973). The thin-walled, narrow-bore arterial catheters then in use were, however, unsuitable, being easily blocked, kinked, or broken. Moreover, when drainage was required for a longer period, the tubes needed changing from time to time, as they became blocked by the deposition of urinary salts. Most authors, at this time, failed to solve these difficulties and although SAXTON *et al.* (1972) had some success with wide-bore catheters, they emphatically stated that "the definite method had not been found."

Recently a relatively small number of patient series has been reported where puncture nephrostomy was performed using techniques similar to the one described here (BARBARIC *et al.*, 1976; BURNETT *et al.*, 1976; HARRIS *et al.*, 1976). All those early punctures, being performed from the back, ought to be regarded as pyelostomies and as such have certain basic disadvantages. Not only were the tubes or catheters kinked or broken when the patient lay down or sat up, but puncture in the region of the hilus endangered the large renal vessels much more than a lateral approach via the renal parenchyma. To avoid these disadvantages a technique for percutaneous nephrostomy has been devised which uses a wide-bore replaceable catheter fixed within the pelvis so as to avoid skin stitches and plasters. It can be performed easily with local anesthesia and will not cause undue distress to the often critically-ill patient. Successive modifications have resulted in a safe and reliable technique which can be learned quickly. So far this technique has been used in more than 200 kidneys in our hospital, and over the past years it has almost completely replaced operative nephrostomy. A preliminary description was published by ALMGÅRD and FERNSTRÖM (1974).

D. The Principle of Percutaneous Puncture Nephrostomy

With the help of X-ray television equipment, the renal pelvis is entered with a fine-caliber needle inserted from the side with the patient lying on his back. Radiopaque contrast medium injected via the needle into the pelvis allows visualization so that a long, wide trocar covered by a polyethylene tube (PT) can be inserted. Careful removal of the trocar leaves the tube in the renal pelvis and a small stitch in the adjacent skin fixes it in position. The tube is changed every second day to one of a successively wider caliber until a Foley catheter 12-F can be inserted.

A guide wire is used to exchange tubes and insert the final catheter. Since these changes, just as the original puncture, are carried out under X-ray television control, they are preferably performed in a department of radiology by an operator skilled in arterial catheterization. It usually takes about 8 days before the canal is wide enough for insertion of a Foley catheter, and during this time the patient requires hospitalization.

I. Instruments

The following instruments are required:

1. Puncture needle—at least 90 mm long and with an outer diameter of 1.5 mm. This is used to inject local anesthesia, to puncture the renal pelvis, and to fill it with opaque contrast medium.

2. Trocar—90 mm long with a diameter of 2.2 mm. Like all trocars it should have a sharp cutting point (Fig. 1a).

3. Polyethylene tubes (PT)—85 mm long with a conical end and two adjacent side holes (Fig. 1b). Four calibers of PT are used; the narrowest, Pe 320, has an outer diameter of 3.5 mm, Pe 350 has one of 3.99 mm, Pe 355, one of 4.50 mm, and Pe 360, one of 4.82 mm.

The tubes needed for the puncture procedure are made in the following way. Under sterile conditions, 150 mm of tube is threaded over the trocar. A firm pull tapers the end of the tube to a somewhat thinner-walled, narrower conical segment, which fits snugly over the top of the trocar. After being warmed in steam, the end of the tube is then bent to an angle of 45–65°. Two side holes are easily bored into the concavity of the tube threaded over the trocar. This method of construction makes the tubes best suited to the form of the renal pelvis, if the conical end is placed at the uretero-pelvic junction. An effort is made to design the angles and holes to fit the individual renal anatomy. The excess tube is removed to give a total length of 85 mm.

4. Guide wires, like those used for arterial catheterization, in three sizes: no. 160 with an outer diameter of 0.9 mm, no. 205 of 1.2 mm, and a teflon J-guide no. 160.

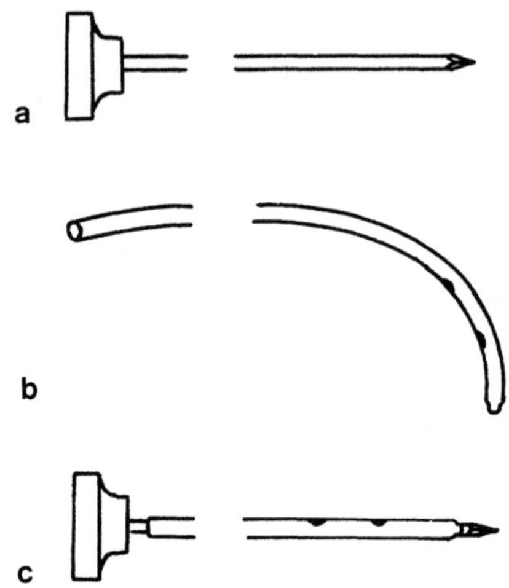

Fig. 1a–c. Instruments for percutaneous nephrostomy. (a) Trocar. (b) Polyethylene tube, two side holes and conical end. (c) The trocar threaded through the polyethylene tube

5. A piece of sterile rubber tube for connecting the PT with a uribag.

6. A Foley catheter 12-F. To improve drainage an extra eye is cut 5–7 mm proximal to the balloon and on the side opposite to the balloon canal. The tip of the beak must be removed so that the catheter can be threaded over the guide wire.

Some urologists are afraid of a balloon in the renal pelvis, for they feel that if rupture occurred, small fragments of rubber might be retained and cause future difficulties. Having used more than a thousand catheters, the authors, however, have never experienced this complication and the advantage to the patient in avoiding skin sutures, with the risk of infection and pain, is considerable.

II. Anesthesia

Percutaneous renal puncture is performed with local anesthesia. This is considered one of the advantages of the method, for it requires only infiltration of the skin and subcutaneous tissue. Premedication, e.g., with atropine + diazepam, is advisable. Even subsequent changes of tube and catheter can, with advantage, be performed with premedication and, if necessary, local infiltration. The monthly catheter changes in a permanent nephrostomy never require any type of premedication or anesthesia.

III. The Technique of Percutaneous Puncture Nephrostomy

1. Puncture and Introduction of a Polyethylene Tube Into the Renal Pelvis

The patient should be supine with the side in question rotated about 10° anteriorly. When renal function is satisfactory, intravenous injection of contrast medium helps visualize the renal pelvis. However, in the majority of cases this criterion is not fulfilled and contrast medium is of no help; then meticulous X-ray television screening which uses an image intensifier of good resolution and high gain is relied upon for adequate renal localization. When the pelvis is dilated, single-plane screening with vertical rays usually suffices, but otherwise two-plane screening is required to accurately localize the pelvis.

The renal pelvis is initially entered with a needle 90 mm long and 1.5 mm wide that is positioned as far ventrally as possible without penetrating the peritoneum. The skin is pierced on the posterior axillary line just below the 12th rib. Intercostal puncture should be avoided, not only because of potential pleural injury but also because a tube lying in this position any length of time irritates the intercostal nerve and causes pain. The needle is directed about 10° ventrally and slowly inserted. To ensure that the peritoneal cavity is not entered (Penetration is usually experienced by the patient as painful), a small amount of contrast medium, given intermittently during the puncture, visualizes the anatomy around the needle point. Should the peritoneum or an intestine be inadvertently pierced, the needle should be withdrawn and a new needle inserted further dorsally. The pelvis lies ventrally in the kidney and the needle is directed towards its probable position. A sudden flow of urine indicates that the pelvis or a calyx has been entered and an injection of contrast medium clearly outlines the anatomy. The needle is now left in position during the whole procedure and its length and direction serves as a guide to the subsequent tube insertion.

A small incision is made close to the needle and a trocar threaded through a prepared PT 320 is introduced (Fig. 1c). As it is slowly introduced strictly parallel to the needle, its position is constantly checked on the X-ray monitor. A characteristic sensation is usually felt as the

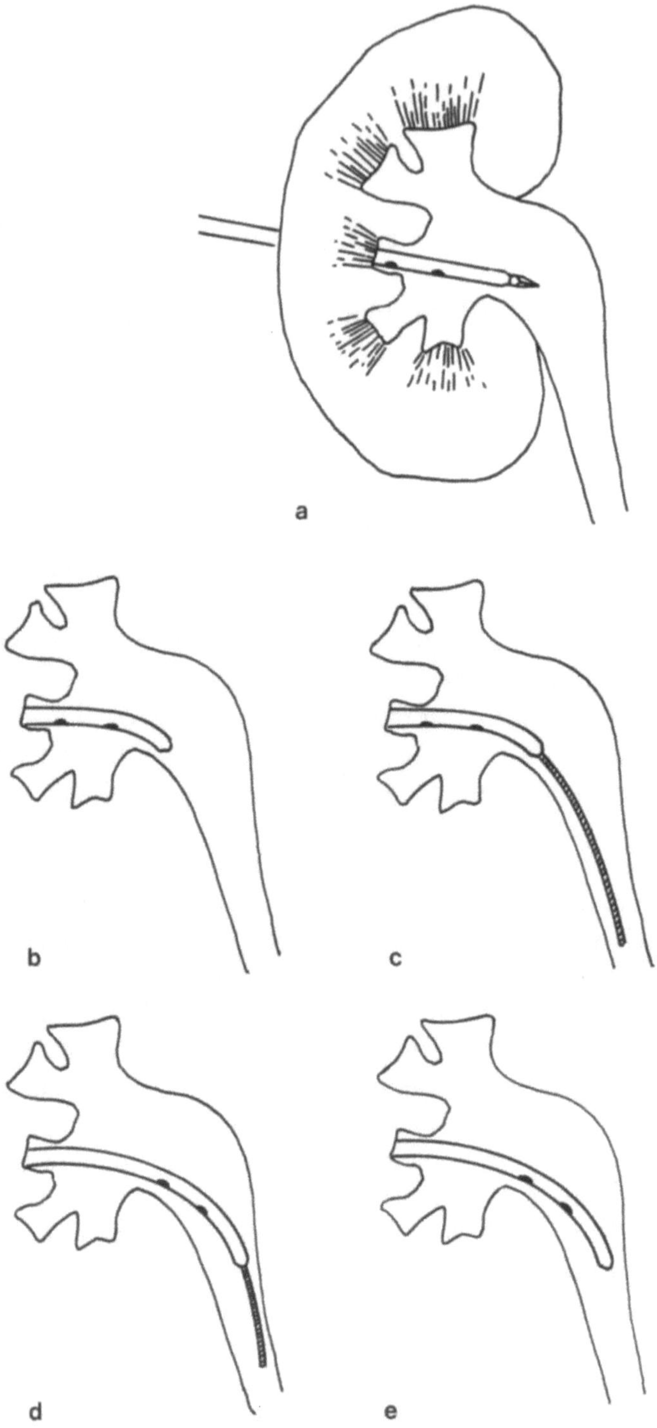

Fig. 2a–e. Puncture and introduction of a polyethylene tube into the renal pelvis. (a) The tube and trocar have entered the pelvis. (b) The trocar is withdrawn. (c) A guide wire is introduced. (d) The tube is inserted until its tip reaches the upper part of the ureter. (e) The guide wire is withdrawn

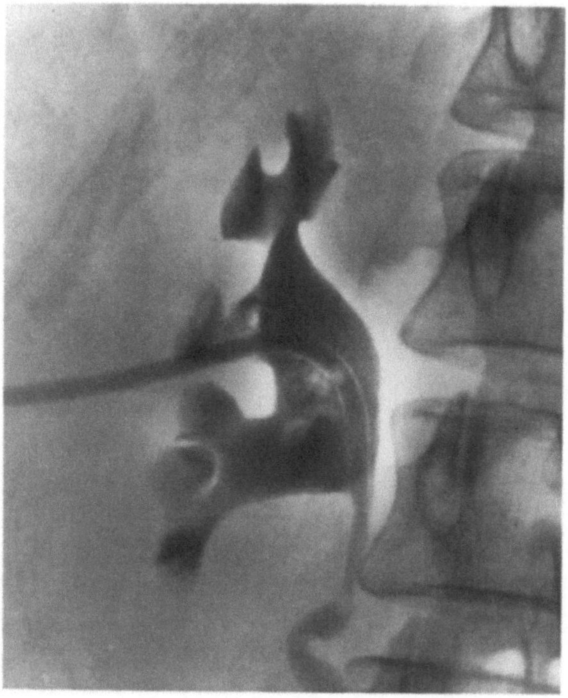

Fig. 3. Percutaneous nephrostomy with the tip of the tube introduced into the upper part of the ureter

trocar enters the renal parenchyma and once again as the pelvis is pierced (Fig. 2a). A flow of urine upon withdrawal of the trocar confirms success (Fig. 2b). It is advisable to avoid emptying the pelvis before the tube is fully introduced or it may easily slide out. The exact position of the tube is indicated by injection of contrast medium. Following the insertion of guide wire no. 205 (Fig. 2c), fine adjustments are now made (Fig. 2d, e). The tube should be introduced at least 4–5 cm into the pelvis until its tip lies at the pelvoureteric junction (Fig. 3) or an upper calyx (Fig. 4). This will prevent it from sliding out of the kidney.

A tube which cannot be directed into the ureter or an upper calyx should not be forced, since its point will often impinge on the medial pelvic wall with consequent risk of perforation (Fig. 5). With the aid of a J-guide, the tube can usually be placed in the correct position.

In the case of a very small kidney pelvis, it is preferable to use a tube without side holes for the initial puncture, as visualization of the kidney pelvis is rendered more difficult should contrast medium leak outside the pelvis.

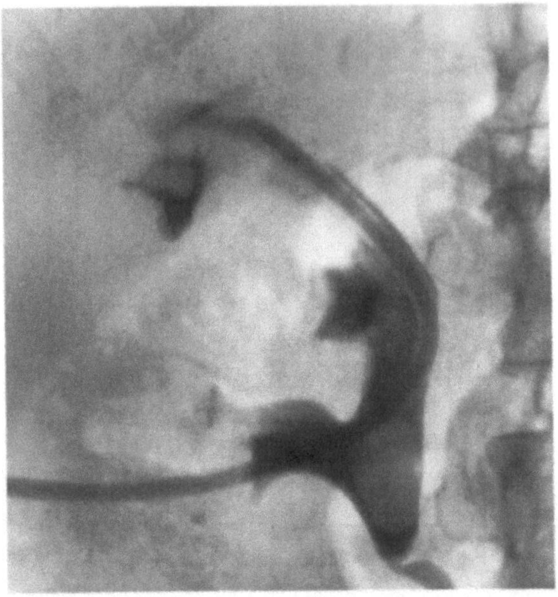

Fig. 4. Percutaneous nephrostomy with the tip of the tube introduced into an upper calyx

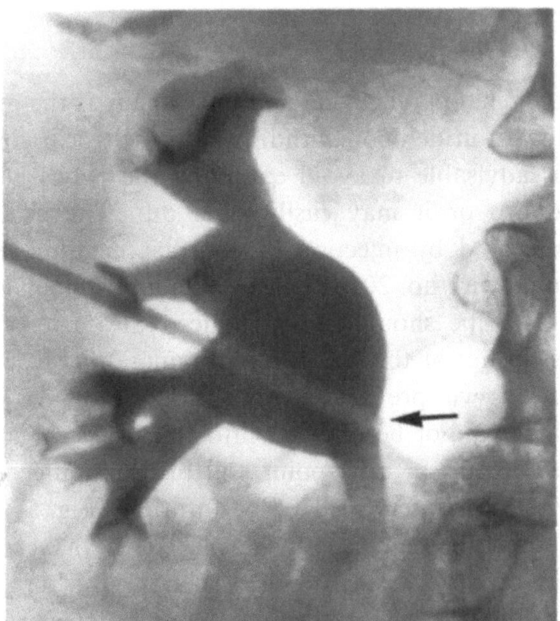

Fig. 5. Percutaneous nephrostomy with the tip of the tube directed against the medial pelvic wall *(arrow)* with consequent risk of perforation

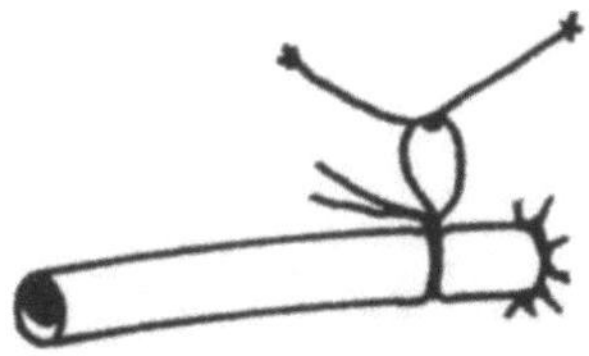

Fig. 6. The tube fixed to the skin with a small stitch

Once the position is satisfactory, the tube is fixed to the skin by a small stich and connected to a uribag with a rubber tube (Fig. 6).

2. Dilatation of the Nephrostomy Canal

Adequate dilatation may be arrived at in the following manner. Tube no. 320 is left in place for 2 days, where upon it is replaced by tube no. 350, and after a further 2 days, by tube no. 355. Two days later the tubes can be exchanged for a Foley catheter (F-12); however, should difficulty be encountered, the rigid tissues may be dilated further with tube no. 360. Exchange of tubes is performed with the help of two guide wires, no. 160 and no. 205, after ascertaining first that they pass through the tip of the tube preferably a few cm (Fig. 7a). This tube is withdrawn (Fig. 7b), and the next in order is threaded over the guides until it reaches the required position (Fig. 7c, d, e).

Before changing a tube, its position should always be confirmed by injecting a few ml contrast medium. Adjustments may be necessary before the guide wires are introduced. The aim is to have the guide wire tips exactly where the tip of the next tube should be placed. If the PT tends to bend and will not pass through the parenchyma, it may be stiffened up with one or two further 205 guide wires. These must, however, not pass through the tip of the tube and must be clearly differentiated from the "leader" guides. The latter must not be removed under any circumstances until the new tube is in the required position.

In those patients where a longstanding hydronephrosis has resulted in a relatively thin renal parenchyma, the whole procedure may be accelerated. By using a thicker trocar, a PT 355 may be introduced initially, thus allowing a permanent Foley catheter to be put in place after only 2–4 days.

If a wider tube cannot be introduced in spite of these manoeuvres, it is wise to replace a similar-sized tube, wait a few more days, and then attempt the exchange once again.

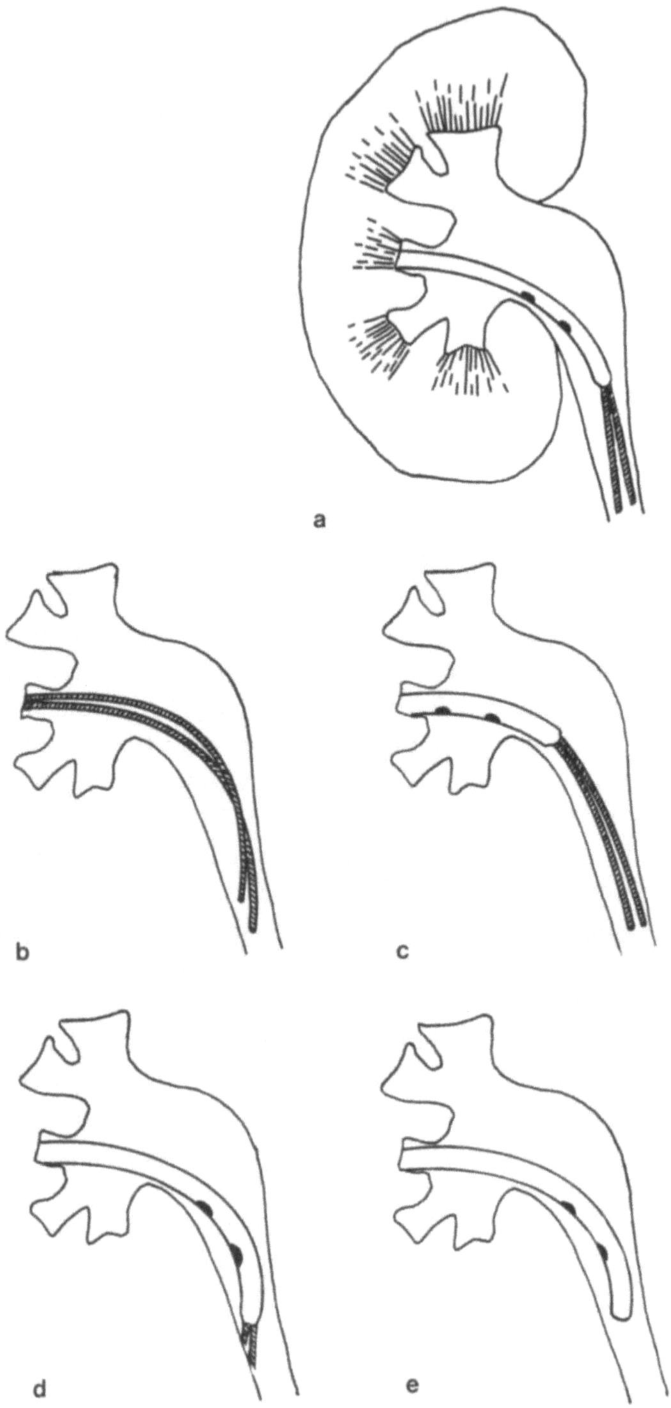

Fig. 7a–e. Dilatation of the nephrostomy canal. (a) Two guide wires inserted through the tube down into the upper part of the ureter. (b) The tube is withdrawn. (c) The next tube in order is threaded over the guide wires. (d) The tip of the tube now in position. (e) The guide wires withdrawn

As a rule, the tubes are changed every second day. However, while changing the tubes the operator should judge the degree of tissue resilience. If resistence is hardly noticeable, a wide, "soft" canal is indicated, allowing daily changes and perhaps omitting some of the intermediate tubes. On the other hand, if a marked degree of resistance is met, it is wise to wait 4–5 days between exchanges. This situation may arise, for example, if the canal inadvertently passes through an old renal infarction or a surgical scar.

3. Insertion of a Foley-Type Catheter

When the catheter is introduced only one 205 guide wire is employed (Fig. 8a). The tip of the catheter is cut off to leave a small hole through which the wire can pass. The catheter should be well lubricated and introduced with a rotatory movement. The guide wire should not be removed until the catheter is in the correct position within the renal pelvis. Further adjustment of the catheter's position can now be made under television control. The balloon is filled with contrast medium and its final position and size checked (Figs. 8b–e).

If doubt arises as to whether the catheter balloon is in the renal pelvis, the guide wire should not be removed but rather an attempt made to blow up the balloon with a small amount of contrast medium. If resistance prohibits inflation, the balloon is probably in the parenchymal canal and the catheter must be inserted deeper. If it is quite impossible to place a Foley catheter in the renal pelvis, the guide wire should not be removed, but the catheter replaced with a PT 360 and a new attempt made after one or two days.

4. Inflation of the Balloon

Correct inflation of the balloon is the decisive factor for keeping the catheter in place. Should the fluid leak, the balloon will deflate and the catheter fall out. If the balloon is filled with 3 ml, inflation is usually maintained for the 3–4 weeks necessary until the next catheter change, but smaller volumes risk a premature deflation. To avoid deflation, it is important that the balloon, its tube, and filling valve are free from air before the catheter is introduced. Prefilling several times with small quantities of sterile water is therefore carried out with the balloon end pointing vertically downward. As a further safety measure the balloon valve is tied. The inflated balloon should be adapted to

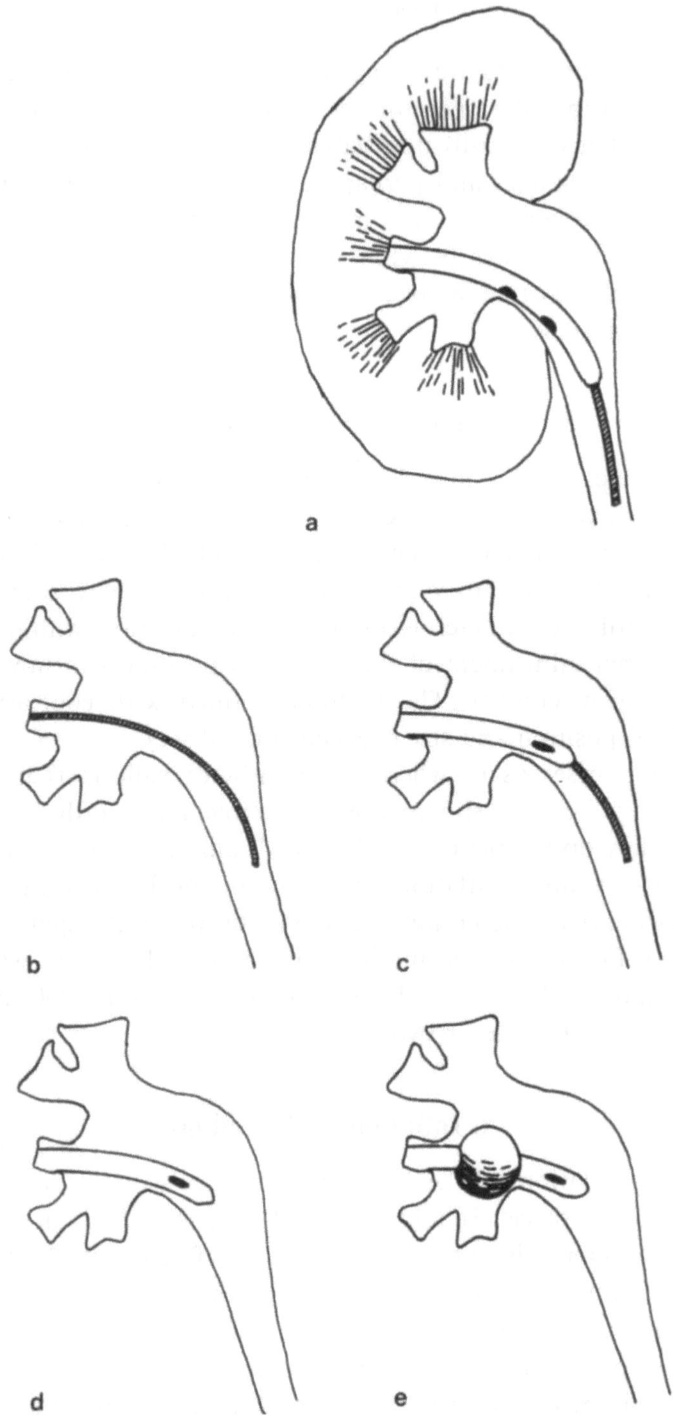

Fig. 8 a–e. Insertion of a Foley-type catheter. (a) One guide wire inserted through the tube into the upper part of the ureter. (b) Tube withdrawn. (c) The Foley catheter is threaded over the guide wire. (d) The guide wire withdrawn. (e) The balloon inflated

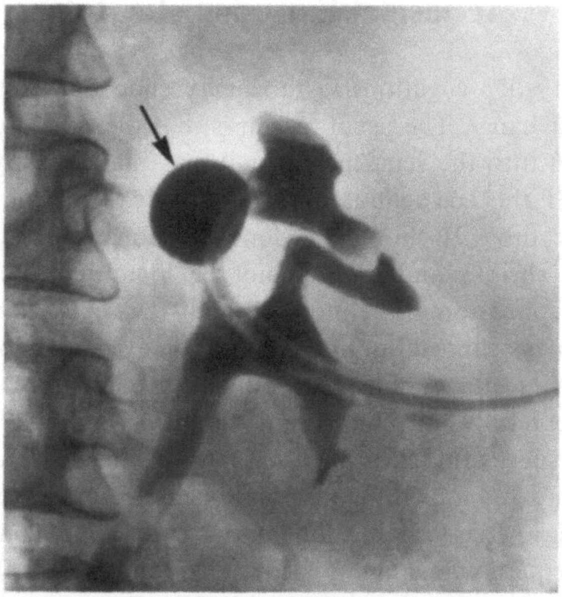

Fig. 9. Long-standing percutaneous puncture nephrostomy. After 3 months the pelvis had diminished to its original volume. The best position of the balloon was found to be in the upper infundibulum *(arrow)*

the size and form of the renal pelvis, never, however, exceeding 5 mls, for an overfilled balloon tends to block out-flow from one or more calyces and is painful.

After a dilated pelvis has been drained for some time, it tends to shrink to its original volume, necessitating correction of the size and position of the balloon, especially in pelvises of dendritic form (Fig. 9).

Occasionally the tip of the catheter presses so hard against the medial pelvic wall as to cause minor bleedings and even pain. In such cases, the whole beak of the catheter may be removed distally to the balloon.

IV. Duration of Catheter Drainage

Before removing the nephrostomy catheter, it is essential to ensure that free passage to the bladder has been reestablished. As a rule, this can be checked by clamping the catheter for one or two days. Leakage of urine around the catheter or renal pain indicates a remaining obstruction. Antegrade pyelo-ureterography via the catheter may be performed to check for a free passage. In the absence of obstruction, the small fistula arising after removal of the catheter closes spontaneously within a couple of days.

V. Accidental Extrusion of a Tube

In spite of all precautions, a tube may slide out of the kidney or even the whole canal. The usual reason is that the tube was not inserted deeply enough into the renal pelvis or it was inadequately fixed to the skin suture. If the accident is discovered quickly, it may be possible to replace the tube. It should be done as soon as possible, since the canal rapidly shrinks and then cannot be identified. The shorter the duration of nephrostomy, the more difficult the reinsertion of the tube. If only the tip has slipped out of the pelvis it may be possible to visualize the canal by injecting contrast medium into the tube. A guide wire can then be carefully introduced into the pelvis under screening. If the procedure is successful, the tube can then be pushed back into place over the guide. A more difficult situation arises if the tube has fallen out altogether. After visualization of the canal with contrast medium and under adequate screening, it is advisable to insert a deflectable catheter-type Selector instrument (see section H). Great care is needed not to perforate the wall of the canal, for this will usually prevent successful reinsertion into the pelvis. If the procedure is successful, a guide wire is passed through the catheter, which is then removed. A PT 320 can now be inserted over the guide wire. If the tube has been out of the kidney for more than 12 hours or if the above-mentioned attempt to insert it fails, it is usually advisable to perform a new puncture, starting again from scratch.

VI. Accidental Extrusion of a Foley Catheter

Extrusion of the Foley catheter is usually due to balloon leakage. When occurring during the first month after nephrostomy, it can cause considerable problems. Reinsertion may be difficult, especially if the patient has had his catheter only for a short time; should this be a week or less, it is rarely successful if more than a few hours have elapsed. It is, nevertheless, worthwhile trying to introduce a new catheter with the aid of a Selector-instrument catheter as described above.

On the other hand, if the patient has had his nephrostomy for a long time, reinsertion of a catheter usually causes no difficulty, since fibrosis in the canal wall prevents its obliteration. It is, however, advisable to perform the procedure within 24 hours, for even an established canal, when empty, tends to shrink.

VII. Permanent Nephrostomy

When it is impossible to remove an obstruction to urinary flow or to perform an operative deviation, the nephrostomy may be left as a permanent procedure. If the contralateral kidney and renal passages are healthy, however, a nephrectomy may be preferred. A permanent nephrostomy is indicated when both ureters are obstructed or the contralateral kidney is diseased. Such a situation may arise in patients with locally spreading malignant tumors of the urinary bladder, prostate, or uterus, and when the patient's general condition is relatively unaffected by the malignant disease.

A well-functioning nephrostomy does not constitute a severe handicap. Patients can lead a fairly normal life and often continue in their occupation, but a catheter change is required every 4 or 5 weeks. Even if these changes are technically easy, they should be performed under X-ray television control to check the catheter position and balloon size.

Non-malignant conditions seldom require a permanent nephrostomy, but exceptions do occur from time to time. A few patients at the Karolinska Hospital in Stockholm have had their nephrostomies for nearly ten years. Renal function is usually unchanged, but occasionally it may slowly and progressively decrease. Permanent nephrostomy will be discussed further below "Indications."

E. General Aspects on the Indications for Puncture Nephrostomy

As long as infection is absent, a ureteric obstruction, even if complete, may be present for several months without total failure of renal function. In a study on dogs, Widén (1958) investigated changes occurring in the renal arteries after clamping the ureter for varying lengths of time. Upon release after ten days, nephro-angiography showed no changes and renal function returned to normal. When the clamp was maintained for longer periods, a reduction in renal arterial caliber was seen to be related to the period of obstruction. After 30–40 days these arterial changes were irreversible.

Similar changes have been observed during nephro-angiography in man. A severe obstruction of longer duration results in a reduction of the renal vascular bed and causes parenchymal ischemia with a corresponding decrease of renal function. If, however, obstruction is complicated by infection, the kidney is rapidly destroyed and septicemia may occur. In such cases immediate removal of the obstruction, or adequate renal drainage, or both is imperative.

The principal aim of treatment in all cases of urinary obstruction is, of course, removal of the obstructing factor. This is, however, not always possible, primarily because of the nature of the disease or the critical condition of the patient. A drainage-nephrostomy preserves renal function until the passage can be restored on a later and more favorable occasion. The faster an obstructed kidney is drained, the better the chance of preserving its function. Since puncture nephrostomy, if performed with the proper technique, puts less strain on the patient than open surgery, the indications for its use can be more liberal than those for operative nephrostomy.

When the patient upon admission is critically ill, doubt may arise whether he can survive a nephrostomy. Since the method described rarely results in any complications and, as previously mentioned, it is not exacting on the patient if performed by an experienced operator, hesitation is seldom necessary. Although the risk of hemorrhage is increased in severely uremic patients whose uremia is caused by post-renal obstruction, a nephrostomy is lifesaving and worth the risk. Also patients with surgical fistulas on the abdominal wall, e.g., ileal conduit, ileostomy, colostomy, are not, in the authors' experience, further handicapped by the performance of unilateral or bilateral nephrostomy.

I. Unilateral Obstruction With Normal Contralateral Kidney

If only one ureter is blocked, it is essential to consider whether the contralateral kidney is well-functioning, diseased, or even absent.

If in a younger individual the obstruction cannot be dealt with primarily, the principal aim of therapy should be to preserve renal function so as to achieve optimal results after subsequent reconstruction. In elderly patients a more conservative attitude may be justified, considering the operative risks. As a rule, a silent, obstructed kidney does not seriously influence survival, provided the other kidney is normal. If a long stretch of ureter must be replaced, the risk of postoperative morbidity, even in younger patients, has to be weighed against the desire to preserve bilateral renal function intact.

If unilateral ureteric obstruction is caused by a malignant tumor, e.g., carcinoma of the bladder, prostate, or uterus, and radical treatment is deemed futile, there is seldom any indication for nephrostomy. The silent kidney will probably not influence survival. If, however, an obstructed kidney causes pain or infection supervenes, urinary diversion must be considered, irrespective of the nature of the basic disease. In this situation, we consider puncture nephrostomy a good alternative.

II. Ureteric Obstruction in a Solitary Kidney or With Malfunction of the Contralateral Kidney

If a non-malignant disease obstructs the ureter of a solitary kidney or the function of the other kidney is defective, restitution of free passage is urgent. If this is not feasible, e.g., occasionally in cases of kidney stones, temporary nephrostomy may be a lifesaving measure.

In cases of obstruction by a malignant tumor, the decision of whether or not to offer the patient a palliative nephrostomy is difficult to make. A quick death by uremia can be more merciful than a few weeks or moths more of an agonizing protracted life with hemorrhage and pain. The ability to make an adequate choice exhibits a keen sense of judgement. Patients free from pain and in otherwise good general condition usually appreciate palliation of their uremia. Reimplantation of the ureter is, if possible, preferred. Even when the tumor engages the prostate or bladder base, reimplantation will sometimes succeed, provided the bladder neck is simultaneously resected. However, in the majority of cases a satisfactory bladder function cannot be achieved and nephrostomy is the best alternative.

III. Bilateral Ureteric Obstruction

What has been stated above is valid for most cases of bilateral ureteric obstruction. In this situation, the question is whether nephrostomy should be done on only one or on both sides. In making such a decision, the probable function of each kidney must be considered, for an obstructed kidney may retain a certain degree of function even for a very long time.

Experience indicates that bilateral nephrostomy is no greater handicap to the patient, than drainage on only one side. It is expedient to perform bilateral nephrostomy in these cases, even in malignant disease, in order to retain a maximum of renal function and avoid the difficulty of choosing the better-preserved kidney. For should the tube or catheter become obstructed or one kidney cease to function, an acute emergency is also thereby averted.

F. Special Indications for Nephrostomy

I. Operative Damage to a Ureter

Iatrogenic injuries to the ureter, usually occurring during surgery on the pelvic organs, are unfortunately no rarity. When a gynecologist has to battle with massive parametrial adhesions, the lower end of the ureter is exposed to the chance of damage by suture, ligation, or division. If recognized immediately, primary measures can be taken, such as the usual reimplantation of the ureter into the urinary bladder; but many cases escape early detection. If some time has elapsed after the operation with consequent ureteric stasis and possibly even fistula formation, edema and phlegmon occur in the area of the lesion. Renal drainage for 6–8 weeks allows resolution of the inflammatory changes and treatment of infection, if any. Reoperation, usually aiming at ureteric-bladder reimplantation, may then be safely performed.

A typical case is illustrated by a 43-year-old woman suffering from menometrorrhagia and dysmenorrhea, who was subjected to a hysterectomy. A few days later the patient complained of pain in her right flank. Intravenous urography showed an obstruction in the lower part of her right ureter (Fig. 10a). Puncture nephrostomy was performed. Three months later antegrade and retrograde ureterography visualized a 10 mm long obstruction of the right ureter, located approximately 4 cm above the orifice (Fig. 10b). The patient was reoperated 4 months after the original hysterectomy, the stricture was resected, and the ureter reanastomosed end-to-end over a splint. The nephrostomy was maintained for another month and then removed (Fig. 10c). She made an uneventful recovery.

Ureteric injuries also occurring occasionally during surgery for tumors of the urinary bladder, rectum, or sigmoid colon may be treated in a similar manner. The following case is illustrative of damage done to the ureteric wall following a transurethral extraction or major operation for an impacted ureteric calculus.

A 26-year-old man who had previously had a stone in the lower part of his right ureter operatively removed developed a new stone at

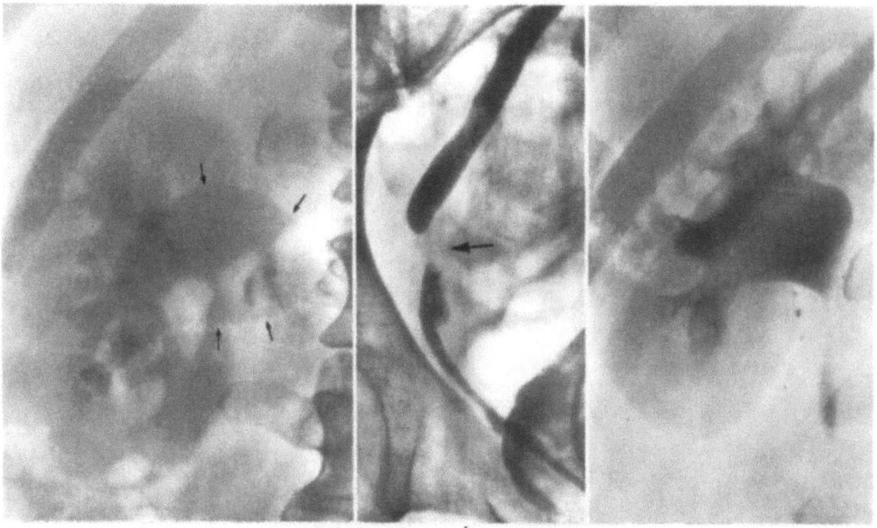

Fig. 10a–c. (a) Intravenous urography (24-h film) 4 days after hysterectomy. Dilatation of the pelvis *(arrows)* and poor excretion on the right side due to operative damage to the right ureter. (b) Antegrade and retrograde ureterography after 3 months of nephrostomy drainage. A stricture *(arrow)* is seen. (c) Normal urography (15-min film) 1 year after resection of the stricture and ureteric anastomosis

the same site 8 years later. After an unsuccessful attempt at transurethral removal, an ureterotomy was once again performed. The ureter was completely disrupted without finding the stone, and so the proximal ureteric end was anastomosed to the bladder. Following a few apparently uneventful postoperative days, abundant urine began to leak from the wound. Ten days after his operation, the patient was referred to the urology department. A nephrostomy was performed and the leakage ceased. Antegrade and retrograde ureterography showed stricture of the ureter with no communication to the bladder or lower ureteric stump (Fig. 11). The stone in the ureteric stump was removed by transurethral extraction. After $3^1/_2$ months of nephrostomy diversion, a new ureterocystostomy was performed which was followed by an uneventful postoperative course.

Less severe ureteric injuries often heal spontaneously, if nephrostomy drainage is continued for some weeks. An example of a minor lesion of the ureteric wall is demonstrated by the case of a 46-year-old woman who suffered from wide-spread irradiation damage of the intestine and abdominal arteries, following radiotherapy for a cervix carcinoma. Circulatory disturbances in the leg required a bypass operation of her right common iliac artery. However, reoperation was necessary and it

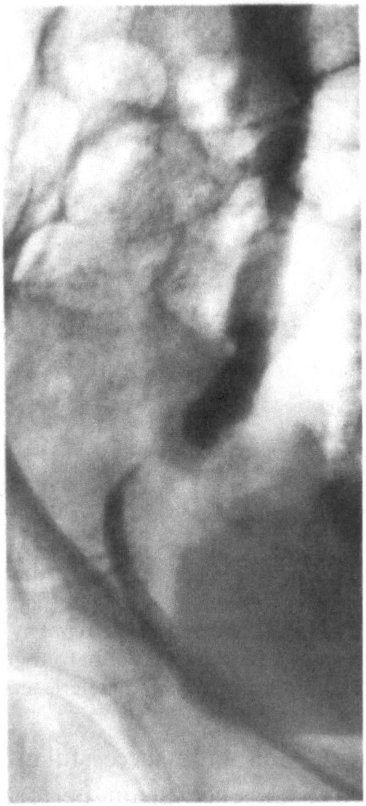

Fig. 11. Antegrade and retrograde ureterography in a case of disrupted ureter. No communication between the upper part of the ureter and the lower part or the bladder

presented considerable technical difficulties. The right ureter was so adherent to the artery as to need separation by sharp dissection. Postoperatively there was abundant urine leakage from the wound and an intravenous urography showed a lesion of the right ureter that was later verified by antegrade pyelography (Fig. 12). Puncture nephrostomy was performed 8 days after the operation. A month later the ureter had healed and the nephrostomy catheter could be removed. An intravenous urography two years later was normal.

The following two cases illustrate compression of a ureter by postoperative hematoma or edema. In this situation temporary nephrostomy allows the edema to subside with restitution of free passage down the ureter.

Following preoperative radiotherapy, a 50-year-old woman was subjected to a radical hysterectomy for carcinoma of the uterine cervix.

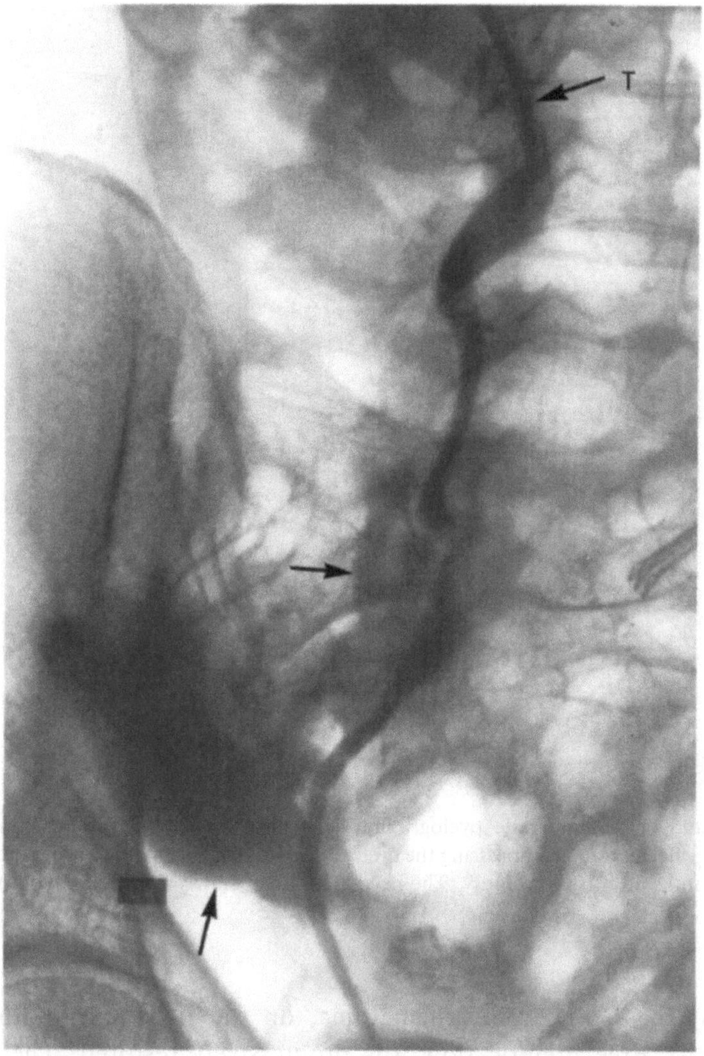

Fig. 12. Antegrade pyelo-ureterography 8 days after a bypass operation of the right common iliac artery, demonstrating an iatrogenic ureteric injury. Nephrostomy tube seen in the upper part of the ureter (*T*). Note the leakage of contrast medium around the iliac vessels *(arrows)*. Some contrast has passed down into the bladder

Tumor growth and dense fibrosis in the right parametrium rendered hemostasis difficult. Two weeks after the operation, the patient developed a fever; an intravenous urography showed right-sided ureteric obstruction. Puncture nephrostomy was performed 20 days after the operation and when contrast medium was injected through the tube, a complete obstruction of the lower ureter was revealed. An X-ray showed a slowly

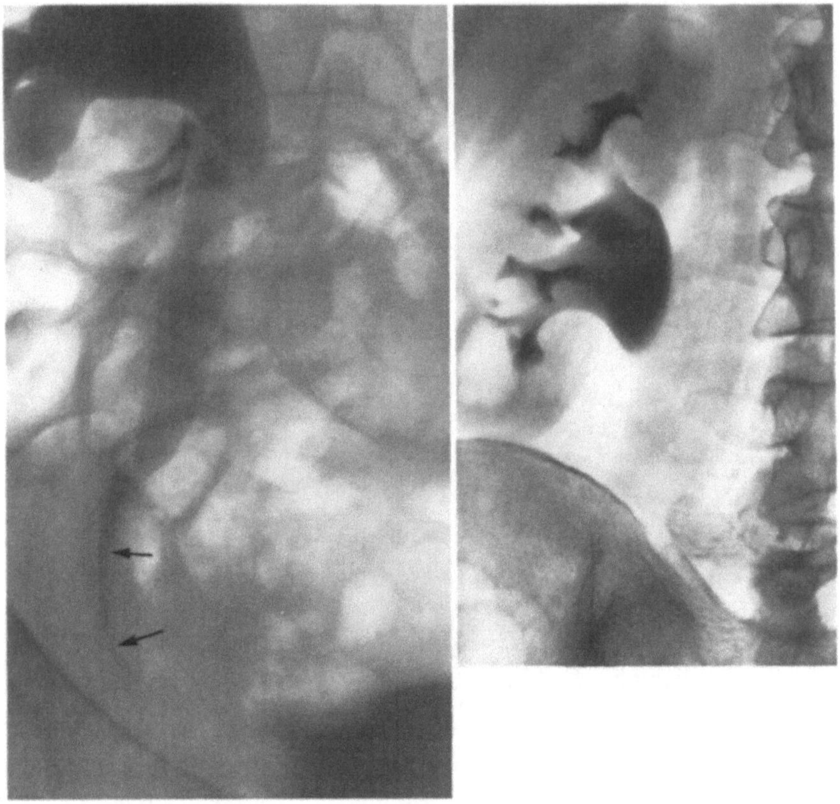

a b

Fig. 13a and b. (a) Antegrade pyelography via nephrostomy 20 days after hysterectomy with a large haematoma compressing the ureter *(arrows)*. (b) Normal i.v. urography (15-min film) 6 months after hysterectomy. The haematoma had slowly diminished with restitution of ureteric passage

resolving mass, apparently hematoma, on the right side of the pelvis (Fig. 13a). Free ureteric flow was progressively restored. The nephrostomy catheter was removed, and the fistula rapidly healed. Six months after the operation no signs of obstruction were demonstrable by intravenous urography (Fig. 13b).

A similar case was presented by a 30-year-old man who required reoperation for an extensive schwannoma in the pelvis which had dislocated the bladder and invaded the urethra. Dissection of the tumor was difficult, and incomplete hemostasis necessitated tamponade of the perineum. Two weeks after the operation, the patient developed pains in his left flank. Intravenous urography showed that the left kidney failed to excrete. Puncture nephrostomy was performed. A week later antegrade ureterography revealed a narrowing of the lower part of the

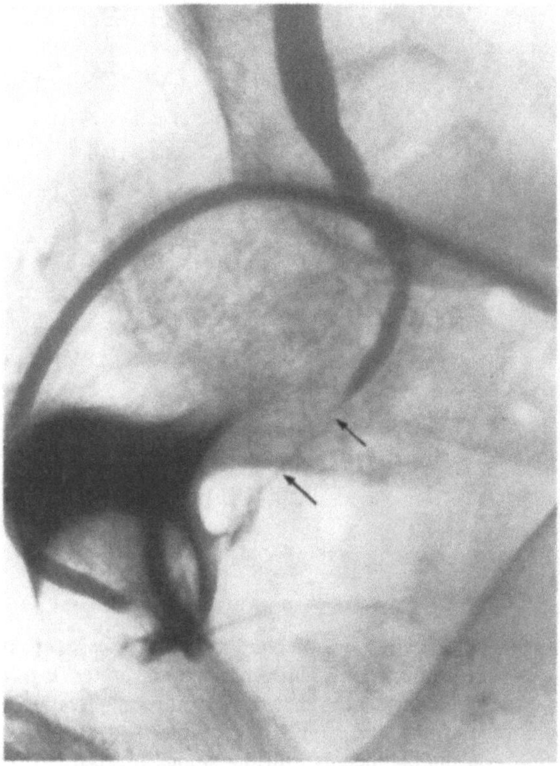

Fig. 14. Antegrade pyelo-ureterography 3 weeks after removal of an extensive perineal schwannoma. Incomplete hemostasis resulted in compression of the distal part of the left ureter *(arrows)* by a hematoma. Some contrast medium passes into the bladder. Suprapubic cystostomy with a balloon catheter

ureter, although some contrast medium passed into the bladder (Fig. 14). This narrow segment progressively returned to normal and the nephrostomy catheter could be removed two months after the operation.

II. The Ureter Blocked by a Calculus

Operative removal of a stone which obstructs a ureter can occasionally be a difficult procedure. This may occur when small stones impact in the distal ureter, especially in obese patients. If, however, the elevated pressure above the obstruction is relieved, such stones, even those causing obstruction of long duration, often pass spontaneously. This is achieved with the help of an operative ureterostomy (ENGBERG and PALMLÖV, 1967) or a nephrostomy, preferably by percutaneous puncture. The ure-

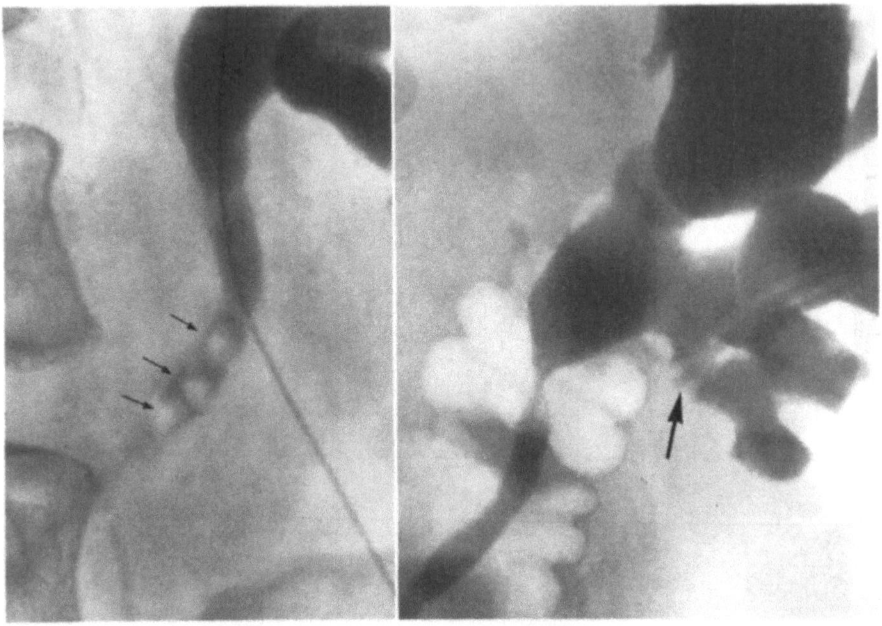

a b

Fig. 15. (a) Antegrade pyelography via nephrostomy in a case of multiple uric acid stones, showing three of them situated in the upper part of the ureter *(arrows)*. (b) Antegrade pyelography through nephrostomy catheter *(arrow)* following treatment with instillation of sodium bicarbonate solution. The stones have diminished and passed spontaneously via the bladder. No further stones are seen

teric wall releases its grip, edema settles and, due to its visco-elastic properties, the wall tends to widen again around the stone and permit its passage into the bladder. Stones up to 5 mm diameter on urography can, as a rule, pass spontaneously.

An obese man, 65 years old, with gout, cardiac arrhythmia, and a previous myocardial infarction had had a uric acid stone removed from his left kidney pelvis by percutaneous puncture (see section H). Multiple uric acid stones later recurred, causing pain and obstruction of the left ureter. Puncture nephrostomy resulted in high-pressure urine flow from the tube. Contrast medium injected via the nephrostomy tube showed several X-ray-negative stones, three of them lying in the upper ureter (Fig. 15a). They were not accessible to a stone extractor inserted in the nephrostomy canal. The nephrostomy was maintained for four months with monthly catheter changes and during this period several instillations of 0.6 molar sodium bicarbonate solution into the kidney pelvis, 500–1,000 ml per day, were performed through the catheter. The stones gradually diminished in size, and all of them eventually passed spontaneously (Fig. 15b). Dissolution of the stones by alkaline solution was here, presumably, a prerequisite for elimination. In many cases of small impacted calculi, however, mere release of the proximal high pressure, as mentioned above, is sufficient for spontaneous passage to occur.

III. Ureteric Stricture Following Urogenital Tuberculosis

During chemotherapy for urogenital tuberculosis, ureteric strictures may occasionally develop that are so tight as to impede renal function. In such a situation, drainage nephrostomy preserves the kidney until secondary surgery of the stricture may be performed.

A 58-year-old man had a recurrence of pituitary adenoma. During the preoperative work-up, his general condition deteriorated rapidly with malaise and vomiting. His serum creatinine was raised (780 mmol/l) and further investigation of the urinary tract showed his uremia to be due to a combination of active tuberculosis with stricture formation in the upper left ureter and a poorly differentiated hypernephroma in the right kidney. A left-sided puncture nephrostomy was performed and tuberculostatic drugs given (Fig. 16). The patient's condition rapidly improved, with a fall in serum creatinine to near-normal levels. Occlusion of the right renal artery with homogenized autologous muscle tissue was performed to devitalize the tumor; subsequent right-sided nephrectomy is planned.

Nephrostomy was essential for the initial management of this complicated case, as more radical measures at this stage were inconceivable.

IV. Retroperitoneal Fibrosis

A small number of patients with retroperitoneal fibrosis, both the so-called idiopathic type and that secondary to retroperitoneal infection, have been successfully drained by temporary or permanent puncture nephrostomy.

A 57-year-old man with ankylosing spondylarthritis and recurrent iridocyclitis had been subjected to a left-sided pyelolithotomy and a right-sided nephrectomy for hydronephrosis, 8 and 7 years earlier, respectively. The obstruction resulting in hydronephrosis had been due to a retroperitoneal fibrotic process. He now showed pain in the left flank, renal failure, and a urinary tract Proteus infection. With intravenous

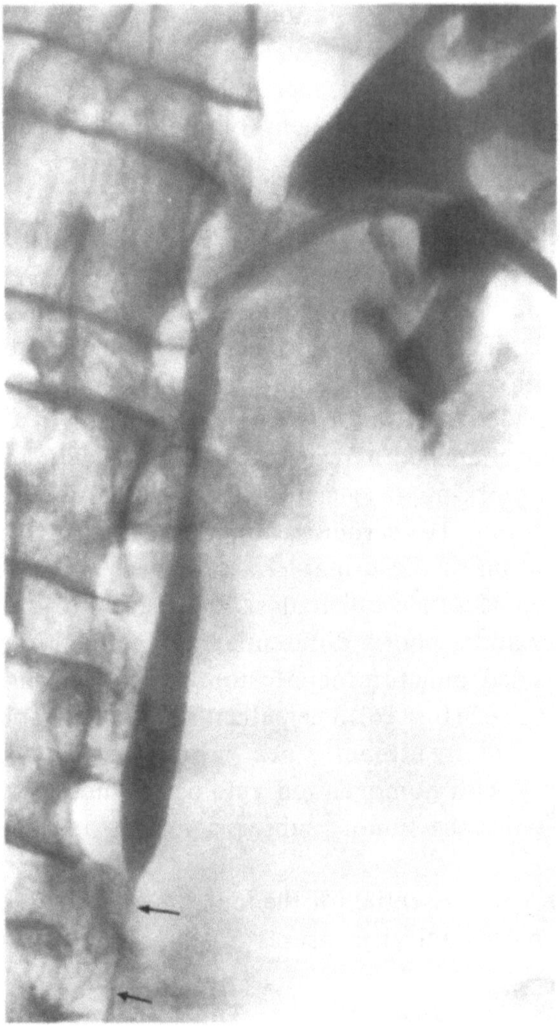

Fig. 16. Antegrade pyelography through nephrostomy catheter in a case of tuberculosis of the left kidney and structure of the ureter *(arrows)*

urography there was observed marked dilatation of the left renal pelvis and upper part of the ureter (Fig. 17a). A puncture nephrostomy was performed and the concomitant antegrade pyelography demonstrated the ureteric stricture (Fig. 17b). Following nephrostomy, the patient's condition improved slowly with serum creatinine levels returning to normal. After 14 months renal drainage the patient was operated upon with lysis, resection, and reanastomosis of the ureter. An area of dense retroperitoneal fibrosis was found, but it was doubtful whether this was due

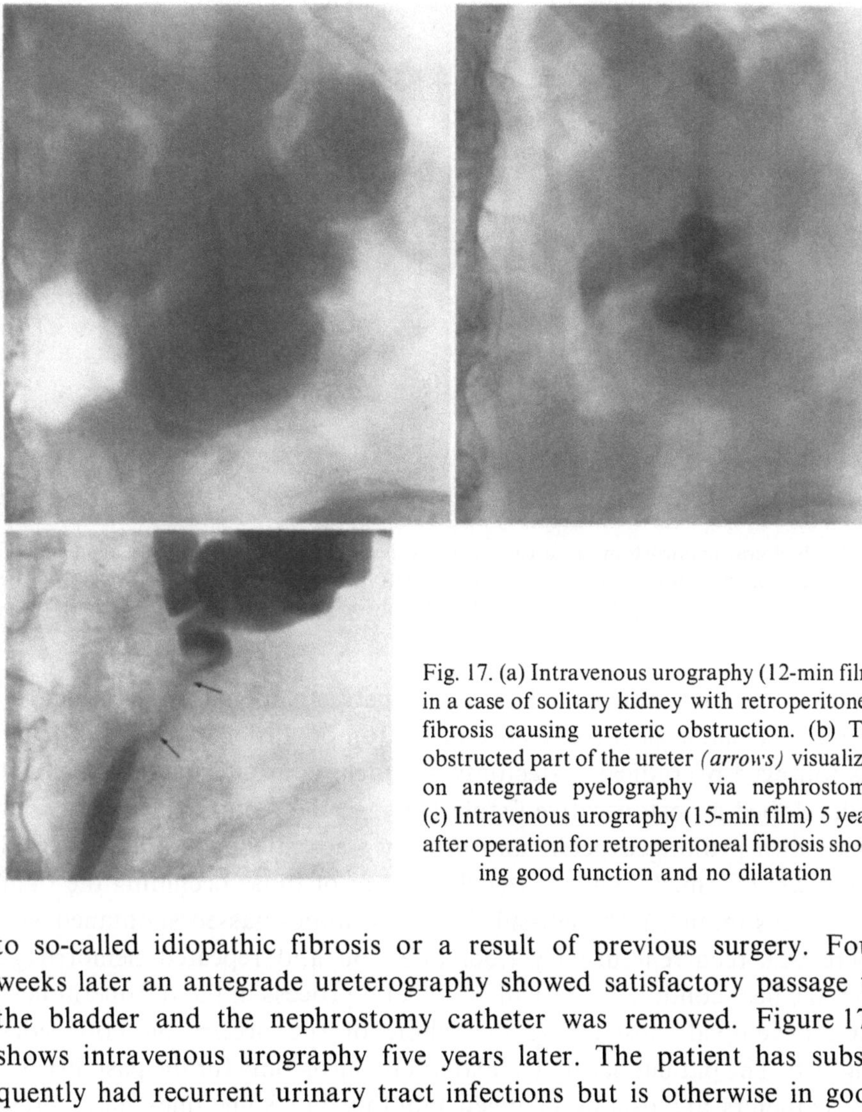

a c b

Fig. 17. (a) Intravenous urography (12-min film) in a case of solitary kidney with retroperitoneal fibrosis causing ureteric obstruction. (b) The obstructed part of the ureter *(arrows)* visualized on antegrade pyelography via nephrostomy. (c) Intravenous urography (15-min film) 5 years after operation for retroperitoneal fibrosis showing good function and no dilatation

to so-called idiopathic fibrosis or a result of previous surgery. Four weeks later an antegrade ureterography showed satisfactory passage to the bladder and the nephrostomy catheter was removed. Figure 17c shows intravenous urography five years later. The patient has subsequently had recurrent urinary tract infections but is otherwise in good general condition with satisfactory renal and ureteric function after 5 years.

Extensive retroperitoneal fibrosis is a very rare complication of urinary diversion operations, usually of the ileal conduit type. A small number of patients who had leakage from the uretero-ileal anastomoses combined with infection seem to have developed so wide-spread and permanent retroperitoneal changes that reconstructive surgery of the obstructed ureters was impossible. They were treated by permanent bilateral nephrostomies and, as a rule, did well. An illustrative example is given below.

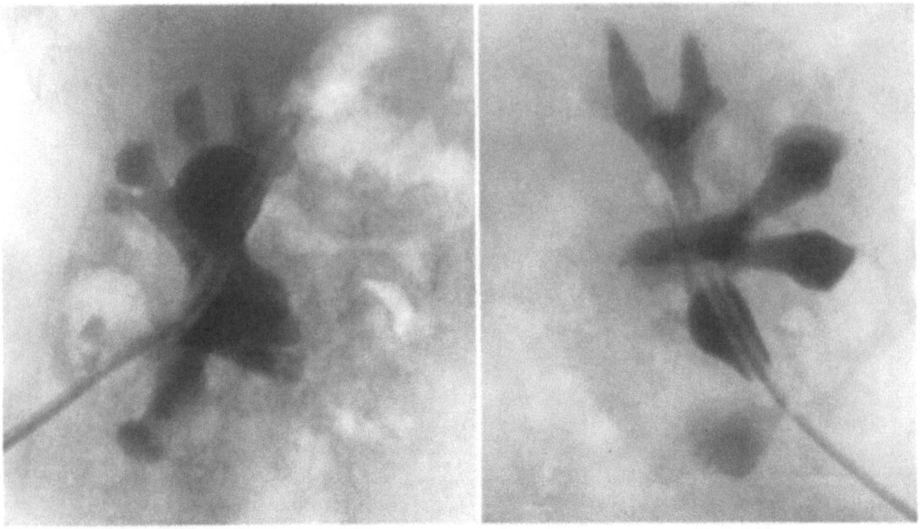

Fig. 18. Bilateral nephrostomy in a case of extensive retroperitoneal fibrosis of infectious origin. No passage down the ureters. On the left side even the confluent part of the pelvis is involved in the fibrotic process

A 60-year-old man who had been operated upon for carcinoma of the bladder had a local recurrence of his tumor. Preoperative irradiation was followed by radical cystectomy and ileal conduit but unfortunately he developed a postoperative fistula between the rectum and cystectomy cavity with prolonged pelvic and urinary tract infection. Bilateral renal stones were formed. While surgical removal of those occluding the right kidney was required, the left-sided urinary stones passed spontaneously. There was recurrent urinary tract infection and repeated hemorrhage from the ileal conduit. Eventually a fibrotic process in the retroperitoneal space developed, obstructing the whole of the ureters on both sides (Fig. 18). The patient has had a bilateral nephrostomy for the past 5 years. The catheters are usually changed monthly but sometimes more often when extruded or blocked by infectious débris. He seems to have adapted himself to his situation and has been able to maintain his usual social activities admirably. In a case of this kind, it is hard to find a suitable therapeutic alternative to nephrostomy.

V. Ureteric Obstruction in Malignant Disease

A 52-year-old man complained of dysuria and hematuria over the past months. Intravenous urography revealed a silent right kidney and moderately obstructed left ureter (Fig. 19a); by cystoscopy a large carcinoma of the base and lateral bladder walls was found. The tumor was poorly differentiated. A left-sided puncture nephrostomy was performed (Fig. 19b) followed by full-dose irradiation. This resulted in complete relief of the left ureteric obstruction and the nephrostomy was removed. Four months later the patient was taken ill with abdominal pains and rectal obstruction due to progressive tumor growth. A transversostomy and additional cytostatic therapy have alleviated, if only temporarily, the patient's symptoms.

In cases such as this with preexisting ureteric obstruction, urinary diversion is often a prerequisite to radiotherapy, whereas in other cases nephrostomy may be performed for the relief of pain from ureteric obstruction.

A woman had had a laparotomy at the age of 47 because of an intestinal obstruction, caused by a malignant lymphoma of lymphocytic type in the small bowel. Intestinal resection was followed by irradiation of the abdominal lymph nodes. Six years later the patient suffered a relapse with diarrhea and intestinal obstruction. Following laparotomy and division of adhesions she once again recovered, but 7 years later, at the age of 61, she developed attacks of severe pain in the right flank. Intravenous urography and retrograde ureterography showed an almost complete obstruction of the right ureter at the sacroiliac level (Fig. 20). Puncture nephrostomy relieved her symptoms, while percutaneous aspiration biopsy from the region of the ureteric obstruction verified a recurrence of her malignant lymphoma. A course of cytostatic drugs resulted in a new remission of her disease.

Nephrostomy as palliation to prolong life in patients with bilateral ureteric malignant obstruction has been discussed (page 145). A rather characteristic case of this was that of a 58-year-old woman who had suffered for 4 months from dysuria and frequency of urination. Referred because of malaise and oliguria, she had a high serum creatinine and was found to be suffering from a stage IV bladder carcinoma, which obstructed both ureters and extended to the pelvic walls. She had been in good general condition prior to her present symptoms and no distant metastases were found. A right-sided puncture nephrostomy was performed. Within a week the patient improved considerably, her malaise disappeared, and serum creatinine fell to almost normal levels. Radiotherapy or chemotherapy was not considered to be indicated. Two months later the patient once more felt tired and began to lose her appetite. She developed facial herpes zoster and a recurrent urinary tract infection

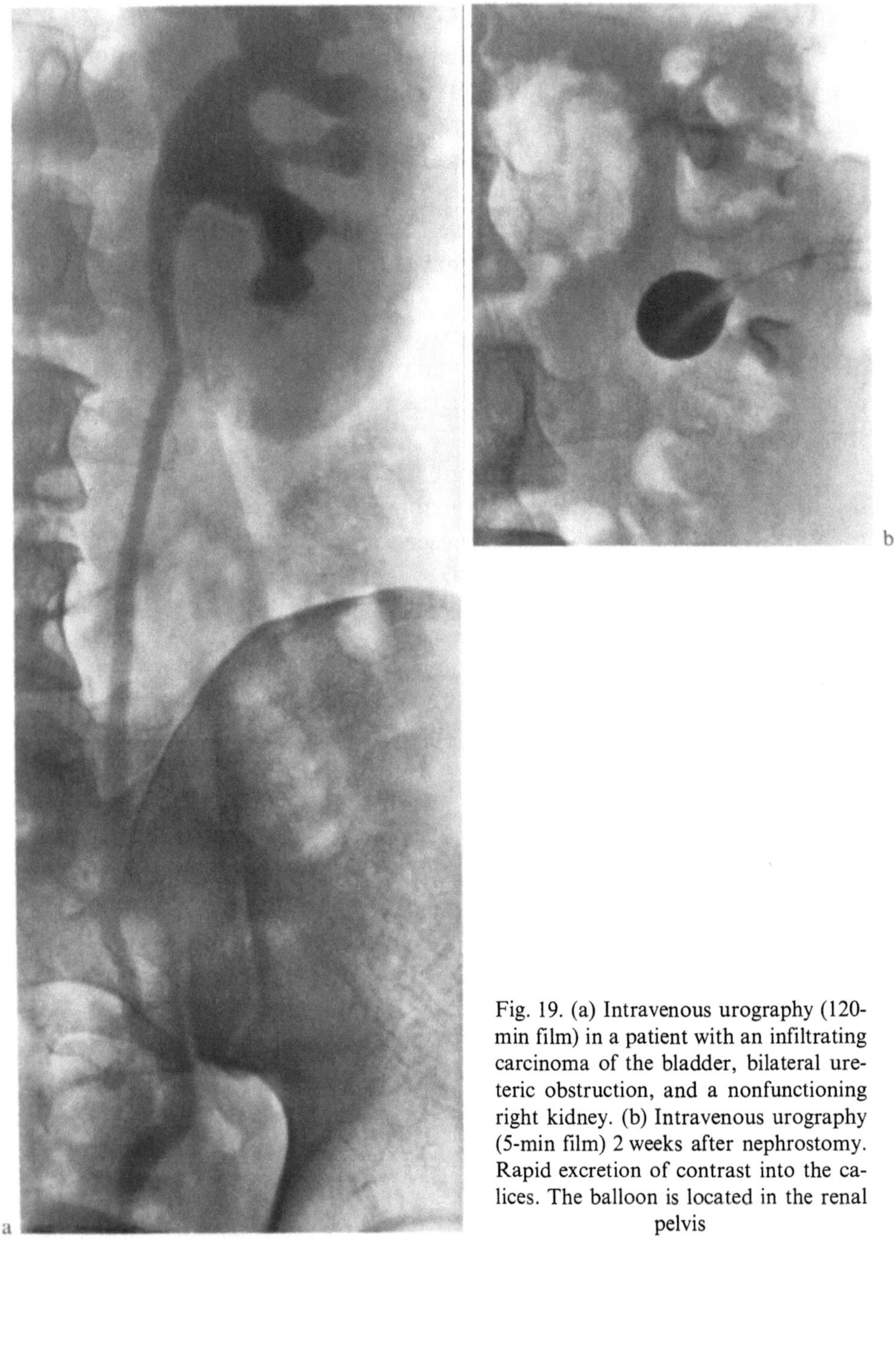

Fig. 19. (a) Intravenous urography (120-min film) in a patient with an infiltrating carcinoma of the bladder, bilateral ureteric obstruction, and a nonfunctioning right kidney. (b) Intravenous urography (5-min film) 2 weeks after nephrostomy. Rapid excretion of contrast into the calices. The balloon is located in the renal pelvis

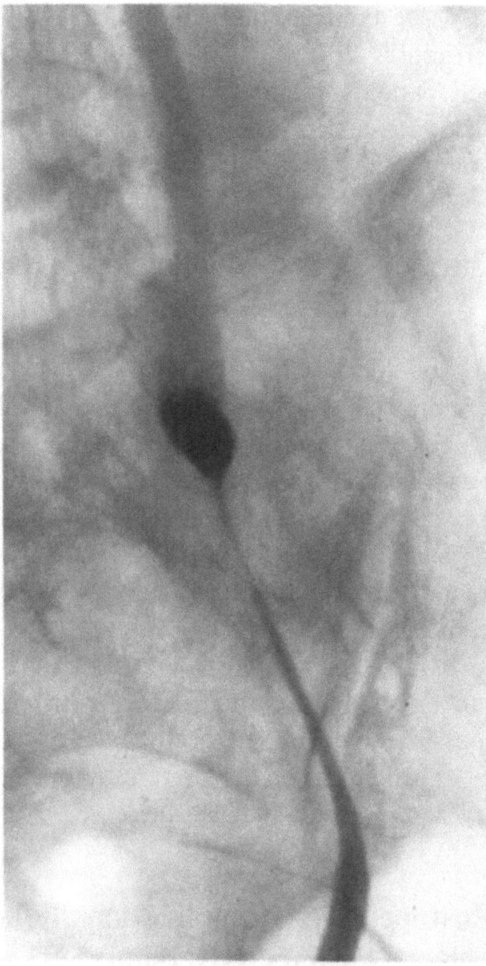

Fig. 20. Retrograde ureterography in a case of ureteric obstruction caused by retroperitoneal lymphoma

and died from her carcinoma 6 months after the nephrostomy had been performed. The last weeks of her life were marred by abdominal pains.

This case illustrates the dubious value of palliative measures in advanced malignant disease. They should be practiced with discernment and without overenthusiasm. However, patients who are in otherwise good general condition and free from pain will often benefit from palliation, provided the palliative measures are not in themselves overexacting. When correctly performed, puncture nephrostomy does not tax the patient and is therefore a useful procedure.

Occasionally the ureteric obstruction is not caused by the tumor itself but by fibrosis following surgery, e.g., for uterine or rectal carcinoma, or by soft tissue contractions following radiotherapy, although post-irradiation strictures do not usually arise until several years after treatment. In such patients bilateral nephrostomy either permanently or as a temporary measure is an acceptable alternative to a bypass operation (ileal conduit etc.).

VI. The Contracted Bladder With Necrosis and Fistula Formation

Necrosis in the bladder wall, often accompanied by fistulas to the vagina, rectum, or both, is a relatively uncommon complication following radiotherapy. Soft tissue changes are sometimes so wide spread around the pelvic organs as to render reconstructive surgery extremely hazardous or impossible. Occasionally the nature of the intra-abdominal lesions as well as the poor general condition of the patient contraindicates preferential bypass surgery (ileal conduit etc.) and bilateral nephrostomy may be an acceptable alternative.

Although the fistulas may dry up, in the majority of cases some urine continues to pass down to the bladder with continuing leakage. It is virtually impossible to effectively occlude the uretero-pelvic junction with the balloon, and ligation of the ureters by open surgery often becomes a necessary complementary procedure.

VII. Postoperative Complications Following Urinary Diversion

When leakage or stenosis occurs in the suture line of a uretero-intestinal anastomosis, such as an ileal conduit or ureterosigmoidostomy, repair is inadvisable before the proximal urinary tract has been adequately drained. The same principle applies to leakage from the ileal loop, a more unusual complication, which may arise in its closed proximal end or side wall and is usually due to stitch necrosis. When obstruction is due mainly to edema or when the degree of leakage is slight, spontaneous healing may be expected after a suitable period of proximal drainage. Antegrade pyelo-ureterography, performed through the nephrostomy catheter, helps to evaluate changes in the degree of obstruction or leakage.

A 61-year-old woman had a hypoplastic right kidney with duplication of the renal pelvis and ureter and a normal left kidney. Because of

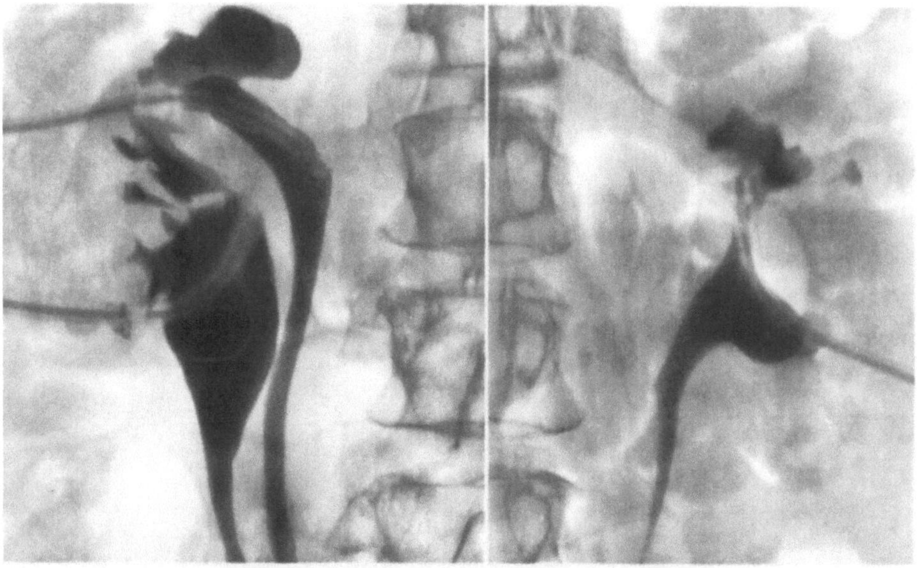

Fig. 21. Bilateral antegrade pyelography in a patient with postoperative urine leakage from an ileal conduit. Right renal pelvis duplication (note two catheters on the right side). The ureterointestinal anastomoses healed after urinary diversion

carcinoma of the urethra she was given preoperative irradiation in combination with Bleomycin which caused an unusually severe irradiation cystitis. Later on a radical cysto-urethrectomy with pelvic lymphadenectomy and ileal conduit was performed. The postoperative course was complicated by leakage in the ureterointestinal anastomoses, circulatory insufficiency in the ileal loop with perforation, and finally an intestinal obstruction. Puncture nephrostomies into the three pelvises were performed (Fig. 21). A minor perforation of the medial wall of the left renal pelvis occurred but with tube in place healed without further trouble. A laparotomy with division of intra-abdominal adhesions and revision of the ileostomy was then performed. The patient made an uninterrupted recovery and upon antegrade pyeloureterography one month later no further leakage was found. The nephrostomy catheters could be removed after a total of 6 weeks.

A similar case was that of a 72-year-old woman with a bladder carcinoma. Preoperative irradiation was followed by cystourethrectomy and drainage through an ileal conduit. After a few, apparently uneventful, postoperative days urine leakage from the wound started. Intravenous urography and visualization of the conduit with injection of contrast medium showed that a fistula had arisen from the lateral wall of the

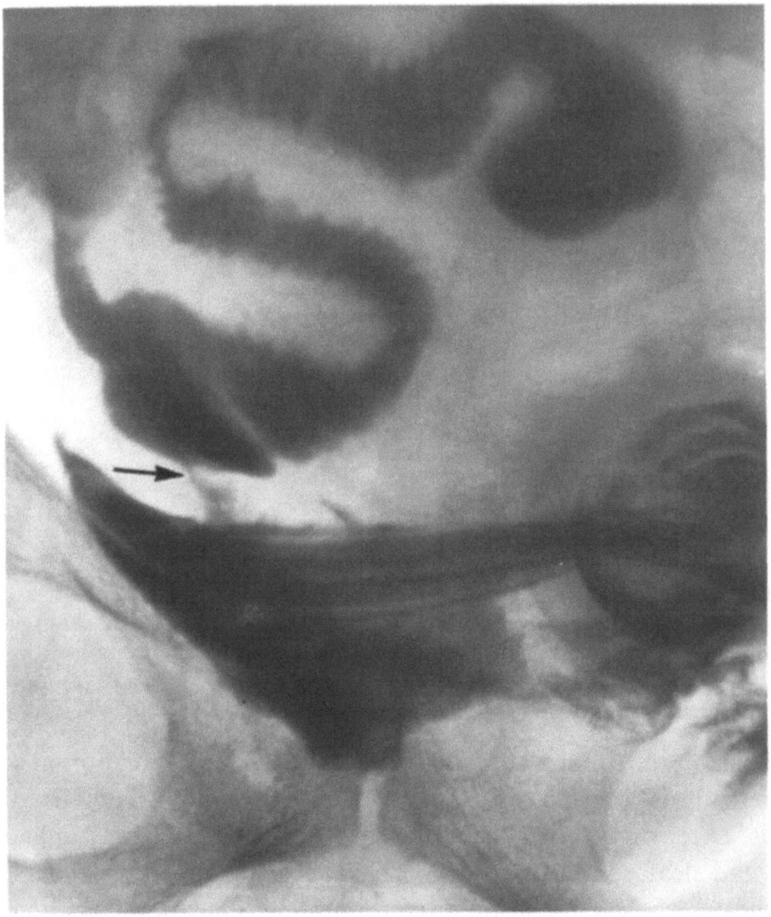

Fig. 22. Contrast medium injection through the ileostomy, demonstrating a perforation in the distal part of the ileal conduit *(arrow)* with massive retropubic leakage

loop (Fig. 22). Puncture nephrostomy was performed on the right side, and the next day on the left. Three weeks later the patient developed symptoms of intestinal obstruction. An injection of contrast medium via the nephrostomy catheters showed the fistulous leakage from the ileal loop still to be present. Laparotomy was performed with drainage of an intraabdominal abscess and partial ileum resection. The patient recovered and the nephrostomy catheters could be removed after 2 months of drainage.

G. Ureteric Obstruction Complicated by Infection

When obstruction is combined with infection, irreversible renal damage occurs after only a few days. Pyelovenous and pyelolymphatic reflux of infected urine within the kidney, as well as oozing of urine through the pelvic and ureteric walls to the blood stream, may give rise to septicemia. High-dosage intravenous chemotherapy, in some cases supplemented by treatment for shock, should precede operative removal of the obstruction. If the patient's general condition will not permit immediate surgery, a temporary nephrostomy may be advisable. Drainage of the obstructed kidney usually rapidly improves the patient and the obstruction can be safely removed secondarily, or may, in the case of small calculi, resolve spontaneously.

There is no danger in percutaneous puncture of a closed, infected pelvis; on the contrary, the temperature falls, and the patient's general condition improves considerably. Occasionally, however, pyonephrosis had caused such massive renal damge, that delayed nephrectomy was necessary.

H. Removal of Renal Calculi by Percutaneous Renal Puncture

On the basis of the technique devised for percutaneous puncture nephrostomy, it has been possible in a few cases to remove renal calculi by percutaneous extraction (FERNSTRÖM and JOHANSSON, 1976). The method shows some similarities to that used for removal of retained stones in the bile ducts (BURHENNE, 1973).

Although not recommended as routine, the method is useful in special circumstances, e.g., when one or more previous operations have resulted in gross fibrosis around the pelvis, or for patients on whom surgery is considered ill-advised because of cardiac or pulmonary disease. Although a stone of 20 mm diameter has been successfully removed, the method is generally suitable for smaller calculi. The technique is similar to that used for nephrostomy, but as a rule the canal must be dilated much more. For this purpose polyethylene tubes 380 (diameter 5.95 mm) and 390 (diameter 6.86 mm), as well as Nelaton or Tiemann catheters have been used. The final catheter ought to have nearly the same outer diameter as the stone and be retained for not less than two weeks, possibly even 4–5 weeks, so that firmer canal walls can develop. However, it should not be forgotten that some of the instruments used for extraction may require an even wider canal. Stones of diameter 4–5 mm greater than the canal width have been successfully extracted, but the technical difficulties involved make such attempts unadvisable. Ordinary premedication can be supplemented by local anesthetic infiltration around the canal so that general anesthesia is not required.

Calculus extraction is performed under X-ray television control with the help of an instrument adapted to the size and position of the stone. The following instruments have been found useful:

1. A Selector-type instrument with a deflectable catheter, sufficiently wide for the passage of nos. 1 and 2 Dormia stone baskets (same instrument as used for non-operative removal of retained biliary stones).[1]
2. Renal pelvis extraction forceps (Randall forceps).[2]
3. Stone removal forceps with adjustable shafts.[3]
4. Specially manufactured, malleable silver scoops (Fig. 23). The scoops can draw the stone from a calyx into the confluent pelvis where it may be extracted using stone removal forceps or a Dormia basket.

Following successful extraction, a nephrostomy catheter is introduced to drain the kidney. Difficulty is sometimes encountered in inserting the catheter, usually due to canal wall damage during stone extraction. It is therefore advisable to have a thin guide wire (160 teflon-coated) in the canal and pelvis during the whole procedure to guide the catheter to the correct position. Following subsequent removal of the catheter, spontaneous and rapid closure of the canal occurs.

The technique is well illustrated by the following cases:

Case 1. A 52-year-old man had severe respiratory failure due to pulmonary tuberculosis. He had been disabled by constant pain in his right flank for three years before he was referred to a neurosurgical department for surgical treatment of his pain. Upon urography an 8 × 6 mm stone was seen in an upper peripheral calyx of the right kidney (Fig. 24a and b). Because of its peripheral location it was thought an improbable cause of the severe pain, but, nevertheless, it was decided to remove the stone before pain surgery was performed. Due to the patient's pulmonary disease, an attempt at percutaneous stone extraction was planned.

Puncture nephrostomy was performed using the ordinary technique. The first extraction attempt 6 days later was unsuccessful, but after a further 13 days the stone could be removed. The technique used was as follows: with the patient in the prone position a puncture needle

[1] SH-4 Control Handle, Medi-Tech Division, Cooper, Scientific Corporation, 372 Main Street, Watertown, Mass. 02172. USA.

[2] 317-1-7, The Genito Urinary MFG Co, LTD, 28a, 33 & 34 Devonshire Street, London W.1. Great Britain.

[3] Universal Nieren- und Gallensteinzange, Modell Pfau, B. Braun Melsungen AG, PO Box 110, 3508 Melsungen, Federal Republic of Germany.

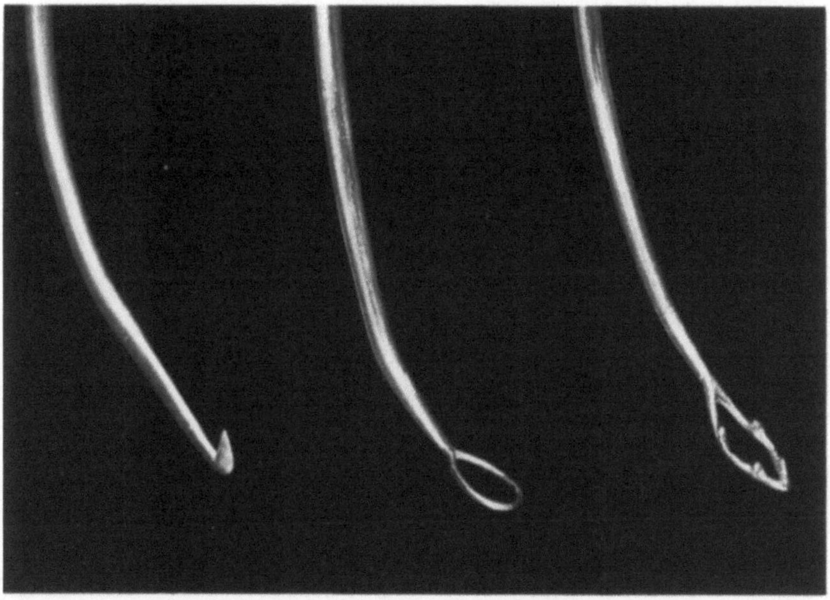

Fig. 23. The tips of three different malleable silver scoops

was inserted from behind and directed against the stone. It was thus possible to dislodge the stone into a major calyx, and with the aid of first a Zeiss sling and then a scoop, introduced through the nephrostomy canal, the stone could be moved further into the confluent part of the pelvis. A Dormia basket was now used to snare the stone. Removal from the kidney was successful, but the stone slipped out of the basket in the layers of the abdominal wall. It was, however, finally removed rather easily by using a foreign-body forceps. A Foley catheter F-12 was inserted but was removed 2 days later. Relieved of his pain, the patient resumed work as a driving-school instructor and is still pain free three years later.

Case 2. An obese 65-year-old man with a history of recent myocardial infarction, cardiac arrythmia, and gout had had left renal colic, due to a 20×10 mm stone obstructing the proximal part of the ureter (Fig. 25). Because the patient was in a rather poor general condition, an attempt at percutaneous extraction was decided upon.

Puncture nephrostomy was performed in the usual manner and the canal dilated. After 13 days an extraction attempt was unsuccessful. But when the procedure was repeated on the following day, the stone was removed. The successful attempt was commenced by introducing a Dor-

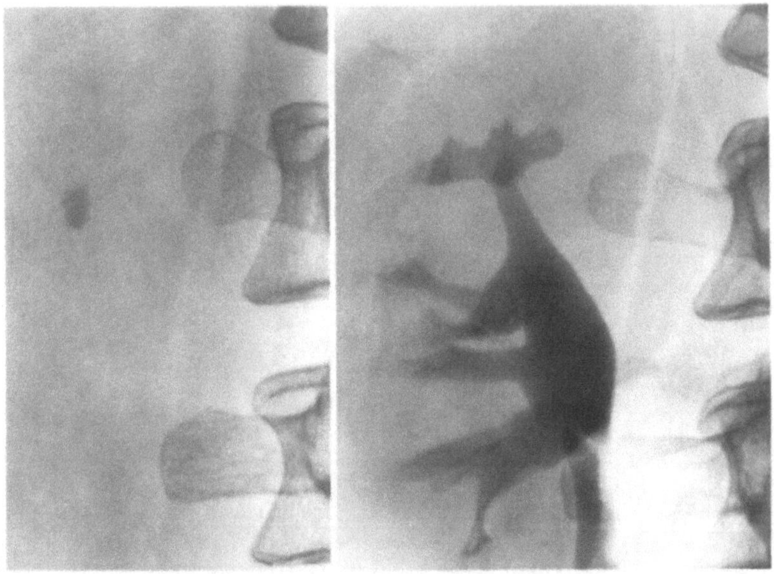

a b

Fig. 24a and b. Plain film and intravenous urography in case 1. Small stone in an upper medial calyx of the right kidney

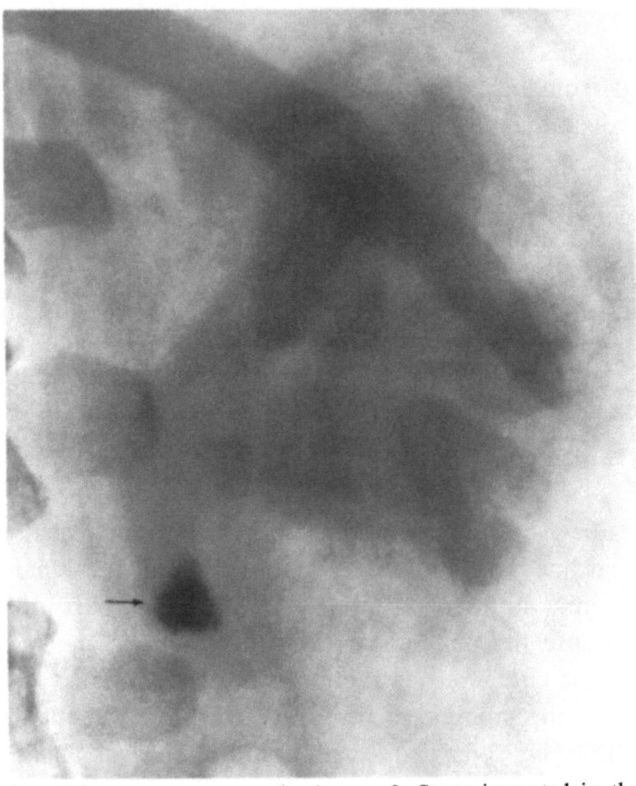

Fig. 25. Prolonged intravenous urography in case 2. Stone impacted in the upper ureter *(arrow)*. Weak contrast filling of the dilated pelvis

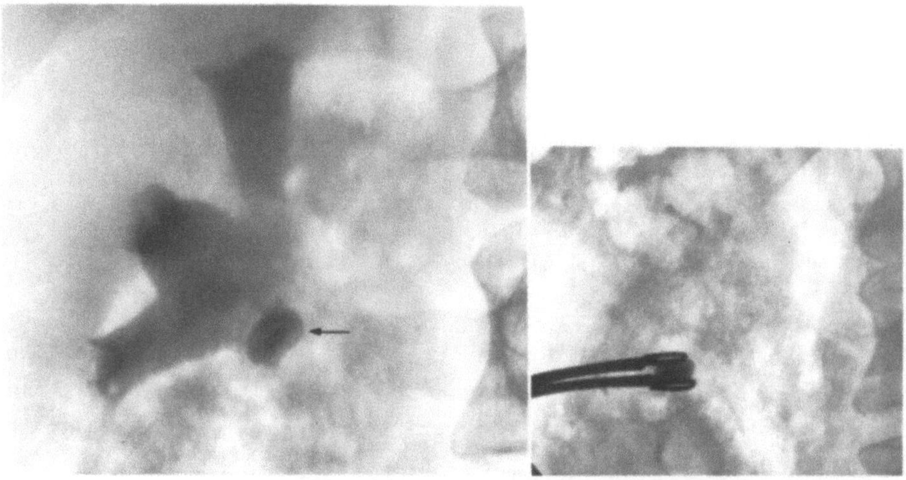

a b

Fig. 26. (a) Intravenous urography in case 3. Stone at the ureteropelvic junction *(arrow)*. (b) Removal of the stone

mia basket, which, however, failed to snare the stone. The stone was grasped with an extraction forceps (Randall) and removed from the kidney. In the perirenal tissue it slipped out of the forceps' grasp no less than four times before finally being extracted. As it was now found impossible to insert a new catheter into the kidney via the same canal, a puncture needle was inserted and the pelvis was filled with contrast medium. There appeared to be normal passage into and down the ureter; therefore further attempts to insert a new nephrostomy catheter were considered unnecessary. The stone was composed mainly of uric acid.

After the patient had an attack of renal colic on the same side a week later, intravenous urography showed obstructing uric acid stones lower down in the ureter. These stones passed spontaneously following renewed puncture nephrostomy and prolonged instillation of sodium bicarbonate solution (see section F, II).

Case 3. A man of 35 had been subjected to repeated surgery of the right kidney for hydronephrosis and recurrent calculi. He now had a recurrent right renal stone, 11 × 7 mm (Fig. 26a). Because the patient was known to have perirenal fibrosis, a percutaneous stone extraction was considered desirable. Puncture nephrostomy was performed with subsequent dilatation of the canal to receive a Foley catheter F-20. After 5 weeks the stone could be removed by using the Randall extraction forceps (Fig. 26b), after attempts with a Dormia basket had failed. A Foley catheter F-14 was finally inserted and left in place for 2 days.

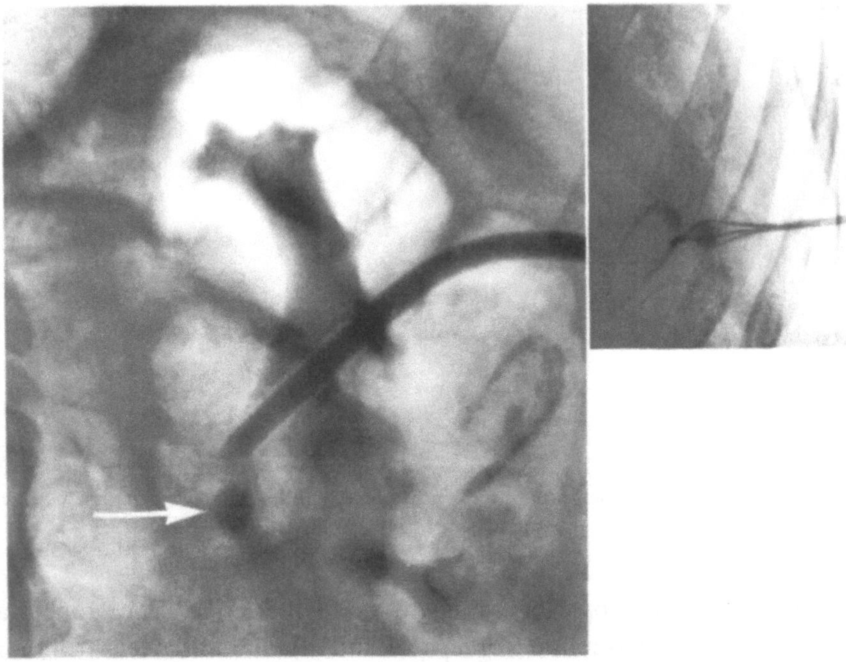

Fig. 27. (a) Antegrade pyelography through the nephrostomy tube. The stone *(arrow)* is located close to the tip of the tube. (b) Removal of the stone with a Dormia basket

Case 4. A 38-year-old man had a recurrent stone, 8 × 6 mm, in the left kidney, seven months after surgical removal of a similar stone in the same kidney (Fig. 27a). Because of the location and size of the stone, it was considered accessible to percutaneous extraction. A puncture nephrostomy was followed 6 days later by successful removal of the stone with a Dormia basket (Fig. 27b). A tube 360 inserted through the nephrostomy canal was left in situ for 2 days.

Case 5. In one case the procedure was unsuccessful. A 70-year-old man with duplication of his left renal pelvis had an operation for a stone, 10 × 7 mm, in the upper part of his left ureter. The stone was not identified at the operation in spite of a search lasting three hours. The attempt was abandoned and the patient referred for percutaneous puncture removal. A nephrostomy was performed on each of the two pelvises, and the stone was located in a small pocket in the upper part of the ureter. Several attempts over a four-week-period to remove the stone using various instruments, however, failed. A J-guide was therefore introduced and directed against the stone where it could be used as an indicator when the stone was removed at subsequent reoperation.

As indicated by these case reports, the method demands a good deal of ingenuity and adaptability from the operator and cannot always be expected to be successful. Especially stones which have descended into the ureter appear to be inaccessible to percutaneous removal. The indications for the use of this method should remain strictly limited until further trials can be evaluated. Nevertheless, it causes less strain to the patient, reduces the length of postoperative convalescense, and when performed in selected cases by an operator well experienced in percutaneous renal puncture it can be a useful alternative to open surgery.

J. Complications of Puncture Nephrostomy

I. Hemorrhage

Using the technique described, troublesome bleeding is most unusual. In most cases the urine is clear already from the start, but occasionally a mild to moderate transient hematuria occurs. The tamponade effect of the tube or catheter on the open vessels of the puncture canal is the probable explanation of the rarity of significant bleeding.

The risk of damaging larger vessels seems much greater when puncture is performed from the back with a needle directed against the hilus, than when the pelvis is entered via the renal parenchyma from the patient's side.

In cases where bleeding occurs there is always a risk of catheter obstruction by clots. Regular wash-outs with physiological saline maintains free drainage and the bleeding usually ceases spontaneously within a few days (Fig. 28a, and b). The usual cause of this hemorrhage is perforation of the medial pelvic wall with damage to the large hilus vessels.

Hemorrhage from the renal parenchyma is greatly increased in those patients with advanced uremia (LUNDSTRÖM, 1970, and others). The only cases of catastrophic bleeding in the authors' experience occurred in two patients with terminal uremia. One, who died within an hour of nephrostomy from severe perirenal hemorrhage, suffered from prostatic cancer and was in deep uremia and a very poor condition when the operation began. The other patient, who suffered from a bladder carcinoma with bilateral ureteric stasis, had small renal pelvises and, in the absence of two-plane X-ray equipment, all attempts to perform a puncture failed. However, larger veins in the region of the hilus were damaged

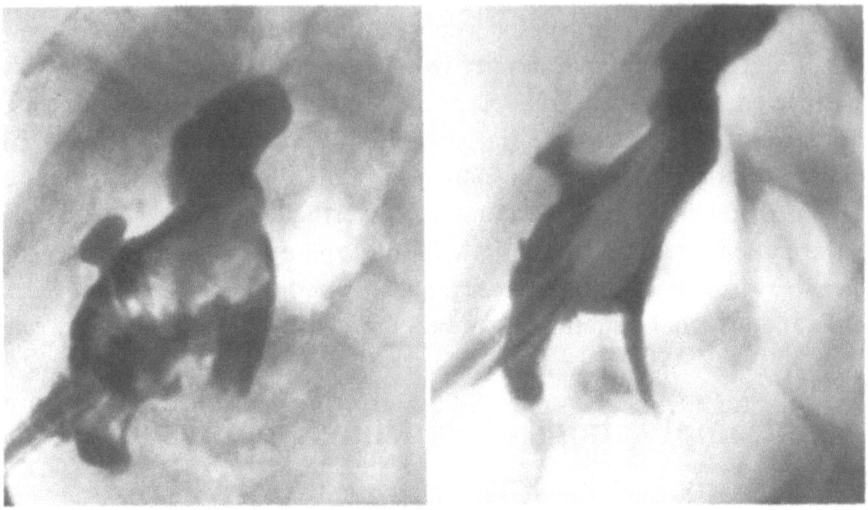

a b

Fig. 28. (a) Antegrade pyelography in a patient with persistent hematuria two days following puncture nephrostomy. The renal pelvis is filled with blood clots. (b) Antegrade pyelography in the same patient three days later. No more blood clots are seen. The urine had now cleared

and a perirenal hematoma developed. Since the patient's general condition seemed little affected by those attempts, an operative nephrostomy was performed 4 days later due to progressive uremia. No signs of continued bleeding were seen once the relatively large hematoma had been removed; however, the patient died a few hours after the operation.

In an investigation of 20 patients for possible vascular damage, a renal arteriography was performed in conjunction with puncture nephrostomy. In one, angiography showed small arteriovenous fistulas at the puncture canal 10 days after the puncture (Fig. 29). The patient had no noticeable bleeding, and his renal function had improved. Three months later he succumbed to his primary disease, disseminated testicular carcinoma. Post-mortem examination showed a smooth canal and no vascular changes in the kidney. Recently we have examined some nephrostomy patients with computerized tomography a few days after the puncture. In this series no perirenal mass, indicating hematoma, was observed (Fig. 30a and b).

Many patients, who died of their primary disease, usually cancer, following prolonged renal catheter drainage, were subjected to a post-mortem examination. As a rule the kidneys showed surprisingly few changes. A smooth even canal through the parenchyma surrounded by a thin fibrous layer led into the pelvis. Occasionally the pelvic mucosa

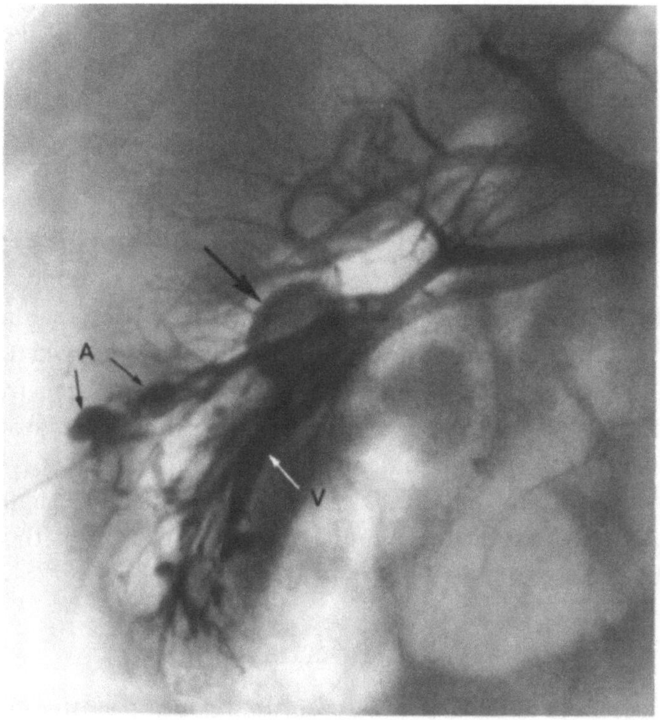

Fig. 29. Selective renal arteriography 10 days after percutaneous nephrostomy in a patient with disseminated carcinoma of the testis. Nephrostomy balloon filled with contrast medium *(arrow)*. Two small aneurysms (*A*) are seen close to the nephrostomy canal. Arteriovenous fistula with early filling of renal veins (*V*)

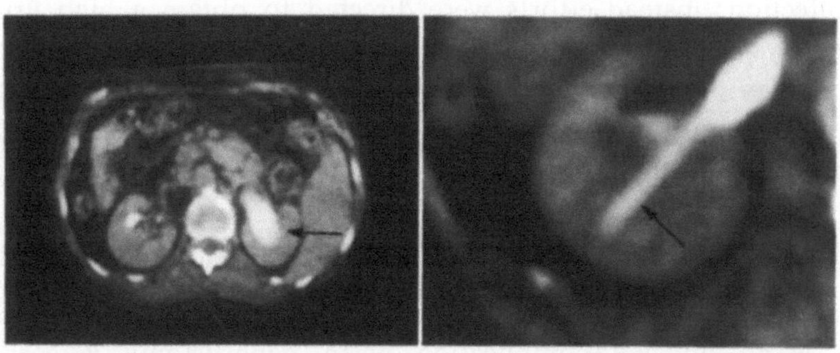

a b

Fig. 30. (a) Computerized tomography three days after a left-sided puncture nephrostomy for bilateral ureteric obstruction. The right renal pelvis is still dilated *(arrow)* whereas the left side now appears normal. There is no evidence of perirenal infiltration (hematoma). (b) Magnification of the left renal area. The catheter is easily seen *(arrow)*. No signs of perirenal infiltration was swollen and showed small erosions where the catheter had pressed against it. The findings confirmed those previously seen in pyeloscopy, which had been performed in a few of the cases.

II. Pain

Pain severe enough to require a mild analgesic, may be experienced during the first 24 hours after renal puncture. Not uncommonly, however, patients describe relief rather than exaggeration following renal drainage. In all events, any unpleasantness soon disappears and when the first tube exchange takes place, the majority of patients are free from pain. Even in the few patients who developed a perirenal hematoma, pain did not constitute a major problem. Once a Foley catheter is in place, no ache or pain should be felt. Distress at this stage is usually caused by inadequate drainage or some fault in size or position of the balloon. These ought to be corrected under X-ray control.

III. Infection

Prophylactic chemotherapy has been used routinely after the performance of a nephrostomy. When only a temporary procedure, chemotherapy was maintained during the whole time of catheter drainage. Sulphonamides, nitrofurantoin and nalidixic acid were the drugs most frequently used, but occasionally antibiotics were preferred. Urinary cultures were always performed during catheter exchanges and more frequently if deemed advisable. On the other hand, patients with a permanent nephrostomy were not routinely given chemotherapy unless they had a urinary tract infection; instead efforts were directed to obtain a high urinary flow, always advantageous with catheter drainage. A mild urinary antiseptic such as methenamine hippurate may have some value for long-term prophylaxis. Acute urinary infection is an unusual complication and requires adequate treatment.

IV. Accidental Penetration of Nonrenal Organs

Puncture of other tissues, with the exception of an occasional bloodvessel, is an unusual complication when nephrostomy is correctly performed. An injection of contrast medium into the retroperitoneal space simultaneous with the local anesthesia shows whether the needle threatens to penetrate the peritoneal cavity and the risk of its perforating the intestines.

In those individuals whose peritoneal cavity extends unusually far posteriorly there is a risk of colon perforation. In one such case puncture had been performed without the usual control. The introduction of PT, change of tubes, and insertion of Foley catheter seemed uneventful, and the urine flow was satisfactory. However, the catheter ceased to function after a week. Control screening showed that the catheter had slipped out of the kidney and was now situated in the descending colon. After withdrawal of the catheter an operative nephrostomy was performed. No signs of perirenal abscess formation or other complications from the intestines or kidneys were found. In spite of this successful outcome, the risk of septic complications when the intestine is pierced must be considered.

V. Inadequate Drainage

When catheter flow is greatly reduced or ceases altogether, the cause must be investigated as soon as possible. Incrustations or thick secretion within the catheter, occasionally seen already after one or two weeks, indicate renal infection. Sometimes routine bacterial investigations should be supplemented by fungus cultures. Very rarely candida may be found in the kidney and may with bezoar formation block the catheter. One patient, who developed massive incrustations and secretion, was subsequently found to have a fistula between the renal pelvis and small intestine.

Regular catheter wash-outs with physiological saline or 0.02% chlorhexidine solution and frequent changes—every 2–3 weeks—will usually solve these problems.

When an obstruction is of relatively short duration, a dilated renal pelvis will return to its normal size and shape after only one or two days' drainage. This may lead to changes in the relative position of the catheter and blockage of its drainage holes by the now flaccid pelvic wall. If the catheter cannot be manoeuvered to a better position under X-ray screening, it should be exchanged for one with a shorter beak or with additional eyes.

A diminished flow may be observed when the catheter slides from the pelvis into the puncture canal, a movement usually due to spontaneous balloon deflation. Correction of the catheter position and inflation of the balloon is performed under X-ray control.

When, in spite of correctly placed tubes or catheters, the expected urinary flow does not occur, diuresis may be stimulated with furosemide or an intravenous infusion of 200 ml of 15% mannitol. Even kidneys which have not functioned for some time usually respond to this treatment.

VI. Disturbances of Renal Function

Diminished function has not been observed in patients with a nephrostomy, rather just the opposite. Adequate drainage results in a progressive improvement of renal function, sometimes to normal levels. A nephrostomy which has been in position for a very long time, however, may result in a gradually diminishing renal function and occasionally a shrinkage of the renal pelvis.

References

Almgård, L.E., Fernström, I.: Percutaneous nephropyelostomy. Acta radiol. Diagn. **15**, 288 (1974).

Barbaric, Z.L., Davis, R.S., Frank, I.N., Linke, C.A., Lipchik, E.O., Cockett, A.T.K.: Percutaneous nephropyelostomy in the management of acute pyohydronephrosis. Radiol. **118**, 567 (1976).

Bartley, O., Chidekel, N., Rådberg, C.: Percutaneous drainage of renal pelvis for uremia due to obstructed urinary flow. Acta chir. scand. **129**, 443 (1965).

Burhenne, H.J.: Nonoperative retained biliary tract stone extraction. Amer. J. Roentgenol. **117**, 388 (1973).

Burnett, L.L., Correa, R.J., Jr., Bush, W.H., Jr.: A new method for percutaneous nephrostomy. Radiol. **120**, 557 (1976).

Engberg, A., Palmlöv, A.: Ureterostomy in situ. Scand. J. Urol. Nephrol. **1**, 63 (1967).

Fernström, I., Johansson, B.: Percutaneous pyelolithotomy. Scand. J. Urol. Nephrol. **10**, 257 (1976).

Goodwin, W.E., Casey, W.C., Woolf, W.: Percutaneous trocar (needle) nephrostomy in hydronephrosis. J. Amer. med. Ass. **157**, 891 (1955).

Harris, R.D., McCullough, D.L., Talner, L.B.: Percutaneous nephrostomy. J. Urol. (Baltimore) **115**, 628 (1976).

Jonsson, M., Lindberg, B., Risholm, L.: Percutaneous nephropyelostomy in cases of ureteral obstruction. Scand. J. Urol. Nephrol. **6**, 51 (1972).

Lundström, B.: Angiographic changes following percutaneous needle biopsy of the kidney, p. 60. Umea, Sweden: Centraltryckeriet 1971.

Molin, J., Ulmsten, U.: Percutaneous nephropyelostomy. Opusc. med. (Stockh.) **16**, 270 (1971).

Saxton, H.M., Ogg, C.S., Cameron, J.S.: Neddle nephrostomy. Brit. med. Bull. **28**, 210 (1972).

Ulmsten, U., Molin, J.: Percutaneous nephropyelostomy in postrenal obstruction. Acta obstet. gynec. scand. **52**, 147 (1973).

Vela Navarrete, R.: Repeat direct pyelography via needle nephrostomy. Acta radiol. Diagn. **11**, 33 (1971).

Wickbom, I.: Pyelography after direct puncture of the renal pelvis. Acta radiol. (Stockh.) **41**, 505 (1954).

Widén, T.: Renal angiography during and after unilateral ureteric occlusion. A long-term experimental study in dogs. Acta radiol. (Stockh.) **162**, (1958).

Author Index

Page numbers in *italics* refer to the references

Subject Index

Urological Research

H. J. de Voogt,
Urologist,
University Leiden

P. Rathert,
Urologist,
University Aachen

M. E. Beyer-Boon,
Pathologist,
University Leiden

Urinary Cytology

Phase-Contrast Microscopy and Analysis of Stained Smears

Foreword by L. G. Koss

321 figures, mostly in color, 12 tables. Approx. 200 pages. 1977
Cloth DM 98,–; US $ 43.20
ISBN 3-540-08042-2
Prices are subject to change without notice

The early detection of tumors of the bladder, ureter, and the renal pelvis is an urgent medical problem of our time. The number of bladder carcinomas is increasing in all industrial countries. The most important factor for the improvement of cancer treatment, however, is improving the means of early detection. The cytologic examination of urine is the only generally applicable, absolutely safe, effective and informative method in the early detection of urothelial carcinomas. The introduction of routine cytologic examinations for the detection of genital tumors in women has already led to an improvement of the chance of survival. This monograph aims to give a survey of urinary cytology in the diagnosis and control of the cause of urothelial tumors. It is hoped that this will encourage similar developments in the treatment of tumors of the bladder, ureter, and renal pelvis.

This atlas should give the practitioner the possibility to make his own judgements with the help of phase contrast microscopy and offer the specialist and cytologist a detailed presentation of the results of staining techniques (Papanicolaou, Giemsa (M.G.G.), methylene blue).

The statistical comparison of examination methods and the certainty of the effectiveness of urinary cytologic techniques confirm the wide range of possibilities of this method for the early detection of cancer. The more extensive application of urinary cytologic techniques, as they are presented in the book, must lead to an improvement in therapy in particular of bladder carcinomas.

Contents:
Clinical Applications of Urinary Cytology. – Preparatory Techniques. – Urinary Cytology and its Relationship to Histology of the Urinary Tract. – Phase Contrast Microscopy of the Urinary Sediment. – Methylene Blue Stain of the Urinary Sediment. – Epidemiology and Etiology of Urothelial Tumors. – Efficacy of Urinary Cytology in the Detection of Tumors of the Urinary Tract.

Springer-Verlag
Berlin
Heidelberg
New York

MIX
Papier aus verantwortungsvollen Quellen
Paper from responsible sources
FSC® C105338

If you have any concerns about our products,
you can contact us on
ProductSafety@springernature.com

In case Publisher is established outside the EU,
the EU authorized representative is:
Springer Nature Customer Service Center GmbH
Europaplatz 3, 69115 Heidelberg, Germany

Printed by Libri Plureos GmbH
in Hamburg, Germany